To wilson.
from Pam.
with my love.
    June 2004.

AN OXFORD ANTHOLOGY

New Zealand Love Poems

Edited by Lauris Edmond

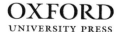
OXFORD
UNIVERSITY PRESS

OXFORD

UNIVERSITY PRESS

540 Great South Road, Greenlane, PO Box 11-149, Auckland, New Zealand

Oxford University Press is a department of the University of Oxford. It furthers the University's objective of excellence in research, scholarship, and education by publishing worldwide in

Oxford   New York

Athens   Auckland   Bangkok   Bogotá   Buenos Aires   Calcutta   Cape Town
Chennai   Dar es Salaam   Delhi   Florence   Hong Kong   Istanbul   Karachi
Kuala Lumpur   Madrid   Melbourne   Mexico City   Mumbai   Nairobi   Paris
Port Moresby   São Paulo   Singapore Shanghai Taipei   Tokyo   Toronto   Warsaw

with associated companies in Berlin   Ibadan

ISBN   0 19 558398 1

Edited by Cathryn Game
Text design by Judith Grace
Cover design by Karen Trump
Typeset by Solo Typesetting, South Australia
Printed by Kyodo Printing Co. (Singapore) Pte Ltd

Contents

Part 5   Our long voyaging   **209**

Preface

Preparing this anthology was among Lauris Edmond's last 'projects'—a word she commonly used to describe the many tasks she so energetically undertook. She died on 28 January 2000, just after the final selection for this volume had been sent to the publisher.

A poet herself, Lauris Edmond brought to the task of identifying, choosing, and at times discovering 'love poems' among the whole canon of New Zealand poetry a generosity that also marked her life. Here, if the reader's experience is anything like ours, are forgotten poems which will come off the page with a fresh urgency, and others not previously known which will earn their place in the memory. Here love, as one would expect, is broadly defined: these are poems in which it is interrogated, expanded, lost, destroyed, given away, and (all the way through) celebrated.

In the last months of 1999, each of us talked frequently with Lauris about this book—the questions of selection, the challenges surrounding any ideas of 'love', the complexity of the New Zealander's emotional map (including that of most writers). We know how much she valued the participation of others in this project. We can name here Linda Cassells, Katherine Edmond, Fiona Kidman, Harry Ricketts, Bill Sewell and Jo Thorpe. A wider group of friends and colleagues will also have shared this book with her, as it was shaped.

It was, however, always true of Lauris Edmond that, although she would explore her subject exhaustively, and usually in company with friends, family and colleagues, her vision was indisputably her own. So it is with this book, one of her last gifts to us, her readers.

Frances Edmond
W.H. Oliver
May 2000

Introduction

My search for New Zealand love poetry began with the principle that each poem chosen must be good in itself, genuine and powerful in the feeling it expresses, fresh and disciplined in its language. And since this is a selection of New Zealand writing, it must be part of the broader picture of how we see ourselves. We are in some ways, perhaps now largely hidden, a pioneering culture, and pioneers need one another. It is not strange that writers here should look to their relationships with others—friends and family as well as lovers—for their most intense emotional experience. After all, as we began our life together here in these remote islands, both Maori and European, we quickly discovered how profoundly we depended on each other for support, sustenance of many kinds, sometimes for very survival.

The fact that such imperatives lay below the popular New Zealand stereotype of the taciturn, indeed positively inarticulate, kiwi bloke does not seem to have diminished their importance to writers. It might have enhanced it.

This had been in my mind, if rather vaguely, in my general reading over many years. I had the sense that New Zealand poets had often been drawn to this most emotionally demanding of genres, and that they had, there as in many other spheres, been inventive at avoiding the direct statement. I began to look for—or at least expected to find—calculated evasions, oblique references, hints, allusions. I was surprised and delighted to find that in fact another tradition also exists here and has been increasingly honoured in recent decades: one of robust, direct, ardent expression of powerful feelings.

But what 'feelings' are to be recognised as love in one of its infinitely varied forms? If a poem expresses grief, or disappointment, or rage, towards a person who somehow could have inspired the opposite (and might have done so), is this an expression of love? Certainly not all love poems are about pleasure. No one could doubt the source of the despair in Sam Hunt's 'Get back to your marriage/Back to your tidy man' in 'Cuckold Song', or of the pain of the final lines of the same poem: 'Forget your grief, your rage/Who you are, who I am.' Then there is the gentle puzzlement of Betty Bremner's 'love was . . . quite unlike the love in books', which carries its own authenticity, recognisable in what the poems says, as well as in what it withholds.

Not all poems that bear this stamp of authentic utterance are addressed to lovers. Indeed, poems addressed to lovers, actual or desired, are a smaller part of the picture than traditional selections of love poetry might lead us to expect. Poets who have never written a love poem in any traditional sense have written movingly of relationships with children, parents (especially fathers), friends, sometimes places, even their country. In order to regard such poems even as possibilities for this collection, I had to ask what kind of 'New Zealand' it was my responsibility to represent here. How have we characteristically expressed our most intense, most secret, most powerful emotions—in a word, our passions? What does a New Zealand context really mean?

But first I must go back to the question of what is a good poem. Controversy rages among writers and their readers in New Zealand over this question, as perhaps it has for educated participants in the tricky art of poetry always and everywhere. I looked for poems with a powerful and honest recognition of emotion, expressed through the rhythms and cadences of language most appropriate to it (in Coleridge's words, 'the best words in the best order'). This is to return to a traditional requirement, familiar to school and university students for at least half a century, that 'form' and 'content' are so inextricably connected that they become almost the same thing. Certainly the authority that makes a poem memorable for me comes from the finest emotional and intellectual balance.

I have read many poems that explored the territory around an emotional experience—a particular weather, a strongly evocative place—but not all were infused with the intensity of that experience. Some lost their way and became descriptions of time or place, with only a vague allusion to the experience that was to give it potency. In the best poems strong feeling is given voice through lively intelligence and skilful and adventurous use of language. As I read, I found myself setting a higher value than I ever had before on this mysterious quality of balance.

At the same time, I continued to make discoveries about the range of experiences that have stirred New Zealand poets into shaping their best work. One must begin with love between adult partners, characteristically men and women (I read many gay love poems, but found the writers had often allowed a generalised political fervour to distort their expression of individual experience); deep affection for friends—a remarkably rich field, this; fine and subtle expressions of love between parents and children. And there is love of place, of one's country. You might well ask, then, how did I decide to leave out any subject at all? Could there be a good poem addressed to a piece of furniture, a house, say? (There could, and is, in Rachel McAlpine's 'House Poems'.) I did in fact say to myself that I would draw the line at poems addressed to animals—and then was so enchanted by Bernadette Hall's 'Duck' that I broke that rule too.

So, the poems were there and in plenty. Now there was the question of how they should be arranged. I considered the two obvious possibilities: the historical and the alphabetical. The second was fairly easy to dismiss. To assemble our poets according to the accident of their surnames might have a certain neatness about it, but as a way of organising and displaying the real beauties of the selection, it would be quite unrewarding. As for placing them in historical order, one would gain insights into the nature of the local tradition, short as it might be, and could note developments in tone and perspective that have come with other aspects of social change. This is valuable in any anthology. However, love poetry is a special field. Answers to my recurring question 'How do we do it here?' might be better found by using another approach altogether.

I began to look through the poems I wanted to include, speculating on the range of mood, tone, and theme. Clearly by casting my net widely, as it appeared I had done, I had assembled a body of work that was powerful as love poetry and rang true by representing an authentic New Zealand experience. It had individuality as well as variety. My perplexity came from the very breadth of this (tentative) choice.

I went back to the principle of balance, and saw that beneath it lay another possible standard—not of quality, but of type: the question of intensity. Experimentally, I set out five possible headings, cryptic notes addressed only to myself. They were: 'Full on', 'Think again', 'Hanging around', 'Further off, the effort of love', and the last, 'By no means'. It felt like a geographical distinction, as though I literally stood on a wide plain, and there were figures close to me, powerful and explicit in the declarations I listened for. Then there were those a little further off whose exact delineation of their experience had found something less direct, more equivocal. Others, in what began to look like my third concentric circle, found some even more complex mixture of acceptance, rejection, or doubt, even fear, regarding the experience of love. There were two more, forming themselves as I peered about; a fourth in which love was often more pain than pleasure, in some way difficult to attain. The fifth category has a good deal of grief in it, and for some reason New Zealanders express grief with great power and frequency. Perhaps distance is still strong within us: a sense of loss that infuses our lives more poignantly than we realise.

The distinctions arose, then, out of ways of dealing with the subject— coming to it directly, hinting at it through other material, expressing awareness of it as joy or grief or loss, looking at it from a distance . . . Looking for these distinctions was a delicate business. As I shuffled and juggled, read and reread, I realised that while listening for a defining tone, I must allow each group a range of qualities, to allow for the fact that good poems are multifaceted. There are many ways for a poem to accomplish its fulfilment.

Thus if 'full on' meant a poem sounded ardent, whole-hearted, direct, its approach could vary from Cilla McQueen's 'I can't think straight . . . god you're nice' to Vivienne Plumb's 'you'll drop into the bottom of nowhere', where the intensity lies in the anguish of the subject, a loved child's illness. It ranged from Fiona Farrell's insouciant 'I am full to the brim with you' to K.O. Arvidson's sombre 'I am the blood that darkens in your veins' in a poem that confronts the frightening question of the cruelty that intimacy can contain.

For the next section I looked for poems that in some way turned away from the subject, as a way of approaching it. Here, too, I must be aware of the complex nature of poetry itself, the art above all others in which the unsaid can be as vital as what is said. Nevertheless, it was possible to separate 'further off' poems from those I found 'full on'. Brent Southgate sets the tone perfectly in his fine poem 'Windfalls'. The sense of direct address to a loved person is still strong, but what the poem actually asks for is indirection: 'let's be more accidental to each other.'

In 'Homecoming' Ian Wedde approaches his experience with another kind of indirection; the physical nearness he celebrates is with the loved person's back, and the poem reflects on love in, as it were, a back-to-front way, speaking of 'passion that needs to move slowly'. Fleur Adcock in 'Double-Take' uses low-key colloquial detail to exemplify the struggle against what she calls 'chemistry'; and Rachel McAlpine, with another kind of obliqueness, suggests that 'Love must change or die' ('Zig-Zag up a Thistle').

The third section, which I privately called 'Hanging around', and which now signals its intent with Jenny Bornholdt's line 'The heart has no corners', moves further in what is essentially the same direction. I looked here for poems that in some way subvert commonly recognised attitudes to love, and was surprised and pleased at the variety of ways poets had found to work in this mode—or mood. This led me to wonder whether perhaps my first hunch, that New Zealanders by habit are inclined towards obliqueness, was not altogether wrong. If my balance is fair, readers will themselves be able to make a judgment on this elusive question.

The group begins with Alistair Paterson's wonderful exploration of an unknown girl writing on his fence, 'Jenny Roache Love All the Boys in the World', and then moves to Harry Ricketts' bluntly worded sestina 'How Things Are'. Here 'if you leave their mother' is followed by 'the likelihood is you'll lose your kids', which becomes a remorseless refrain. By contrast Katherine Mansfield, in 'He Wrote', laughs at the very idea of continuity in love, when she says: 'Little laughs! I see your look/"They Lived Happy Ever After"/As you close the faery book.' And in yet another variant towards the end of this section we hear Bill Manhire saying (in 'Children'): 'The likelihood is/the children will die/without you to help them do it.'

Shaping the outlines of the fourth group, I felt the need to add a new ingredient; marking the movement away from the direct response of Part 1 was not in itself quite enough. If a person's experience of love moves too far from what I have been thinking of as its centre, it surely moves into a realm where the joy we associate with love may be subsumed by the darker emotions of anxiety, disappointment, loss, even contempt. All these are expressed in poems that make up this section. For example, Leonard Lambert's poem, 'The Lovers at Sixty', pinpoints an aspect of this love-and-distance complexity in 'At home the cupboards/are packed with wounding fact/convictions of every possible human failing . . .'.

My note to myself had also said: 'Further off; the effort of love.' To introduce pain, absence, and conflicting loyalties into the experience of love is to risk its dilution, or disintegration; change calls for effort, as Sam Hunt's

'Stabat Mater' reminds us: 'That once I stand up straight, I too must learn/To walk away and know there's no return.' To give a title to this section here, and in the knowledge that often the stance of the poet was far off in time or place, I chose Donald McDonald's 'Time slipped through our fingers'.

However, distance from some hot, heartfelt centre of feeling is not always expressed with sorrow or even pessimism. The poem I have placed first here is Bernadette Hall's 'Duck', a delightful mixture of the absurd and the poignant, while Elizabeth Smither is humorously scornful ('Temptations of St Antony by His Housekeeper') and Murray Edmond stylises his comments on a relationship in 'Go to Woe' as a way of distancing himself from it.

The fifth and final category takes my selection to the limits of distance, disillusionment, loss, sorrow—although here too the subject can be taken lightly, as Rachel McAlpine skilfully does in 'How to Live without Love'. Wonderful elegiac poems have been written in New Zealand, and some of them demand a place marking the end of an anthology that has devoted itself to the complexities of celebration. K.O. Arvidson's phrase 'our long voyaging' holds within it the echo of the unrealised that hovers above many of the poems in this final section.

There were other advantages in categorising the poems according to such qualities as tone or impulse. One was that the poems themselves seemed to react to their context. This is not a fanciful notion. Dialogues were set up; differing ways of considering the love of a son for a father, for instance, if they were placed near one another, created something I came to think of as the voice of poetic possibility. Each time this happens, it casts a slightly different light on each poem. When I saw that Albert Wendt and Jan Hutchison had both written poems celebrating something youthful and sensual—quite distinct from the maternal—that they had glimpsed in their mothers, it was very tempting to invite these poems speak to each other, as they now do. A different connection arose, also unheralded, when I discovered that two poets, Bill Manhire and Elizabeth Nannestad, had written poems called 'The Kiss', which I had selected. Everything about the approach of each poet is in contrast to the other's.

The light, unexpressed dialogue set up by parallels like this gives a double view of each poem. If one New Zealand writer has been preoccupied with this experience, so in their separate way have others, it seems to say. This is at least a glimpse of how our lives in these islands have been evolving.

Similarly, the thematic arrangement can sketch a line through the history of New Zealand poetry. A revealing example is to be found in Alistair Te Ariki Campbell's 'Love Song for Meg', published in 1972, and Normal Elder's 'Love-in-a-Mist', published half a century earlier in 1921. Each deftly moves between the inner world of human emotion and the natural world that is the setting. Each also bears the mark of its time: Elder could use English words like 'meadow' and 'fen' unself-consciously, whereas Campbell writes in a literary environment that calls for a distinctive New Zealand vocabulary.

Yet we can feel the 'New Zealandness' in both, perhaps most strongly in their intense awareness of the natural physical world close to them. In the thirty years since Campbell's poem was written, urban motifs have become more familiar; and in any case such hints as these cannot be an exhaustive representation of a historical process. But perhaps that does not matter. The truth is that some earlier poems, such as Robyn Hyde's 'Close under here, I watched two lovers once' ('The Beaches' vi), published more than half a century ago, sound curiously modern today. Other more recent writers—such as M.K. Joseph or Kevin Ireland—often use traditional forms by choice. It would be a mistake to define the evolution of our literature in simple historical terms.

My 'concentric circles' arrangement also took the emphasis, so strong in conventional selections of literary work in a small community, away from the question of who is important and who is not. The poems speak; not, as it were, the poets. To find out how many examples of a particular writer's work are here, you would have to make a careful search. It isn't likely that readers will bother. Of course, it is also true that some major writers have not been very much drawn to love poetry, whereas writers less significant in the 'canon' sense might have written beautifully in this genre. I have felt a growing pleasure in observing how these effects emerge from the shaking up of traditional anthology patterns.

I hope that you, its readers, will also enjoy the pleasure and sense of discovery I have felt in preparing *New Zealand Love Poetry*.

Lauris Edmond
January 2000

Part 1

This is my voice, saying your name

꧁

Robin Hyde

Escape

Take me, hold me for ever. Tear off all other chains,
The tatters of life that were mine, let them be eaten by fire
And my very flesh be molten, till it lose at last the stains
Of weariness, of hunger, of the long desire.

All that I loved is hidden in you. Presently I shall awake
And draw the blossomed boughs downwards, in the thickets behind
    your eyes;
And the swans shall cry me welcome from the deep-set tourmaline lake,
But the voices of men shall be silent, and trouble not Paradise.

And the sins that were foe to Beauty, these too are known in your heart;
I shall awaken, indeed, and my sword be bright for that fray—
But now for a space of dreaming, the cool boughs draw me apart
And very still is the dusk; for Wisdom hath little to say.

James K. Baxter

Let Time be Still

Let Time be still
Who takes all things,
Face, feature, memory
Under his blinding wings.

That I hold again the green
Larch of your body
Whose leaves will gather
The springs of the sky.

And fallen from his cloud
The falcon find
The thigh-encompassed wound
Breasts silken under hand.

Though in a dark room
We knew the day breaking
And the rain-bearing wind
Cold matins making.

Sure it seemed
That hidden away
From the sorrowful wind
In deep bracken I lay.

Your mouth was the sun
And green earth under
The rose of your body flowering
Asking and tender
In the timelost season
Of perpetual summer.

Anne French

from *Two Love Poems*

I

i

The fields whiten under the moon's
steady gaze. This is a winter journey
we make together, towards the high
places, under the bowl of the sky,
where the mountains reflect the moonlight
with a grave and tender joy,
and the white fields lie open to the night.

ii

How lightly you sleep.
At the first gleam of dawn
you are awake,
turning to me
with wide eyes.

iii

Come to my arms.
Let me show you
how close
lovers can be.

iv

Your face alters
with each passing thought
but your gaze is steady,
unblinking, confident.
This is where
we have reached:
a place of safety and shelter,
out of the whirling night.

v

Now we are apart, see
how little the distance
is between us. At day-
break I wake remembering
your face, your clear gaze.
Listen, the birds are singing.
This is my hand, stretched
out to touch your face.
This is my voice,
saying your name.

Alistair Te Ariki Campbell

Love Song for Meg

It was the way
    the sun came sidling
through the branches—
    points of light
exploding into stars
    as the wind,
eddying overhead
    delicately sprung
the leaves apart.
    I remember most
your eyes and then
    your silence.

Light's undertow,
    backwash of green
from the dull silver
    of decaying trees.
It was the way
    your green eyes
widened and burned black.
    Black and gold
sang the leaves,
    the water rose
in the secret pool
    where all afternoon
I tickled trout—
    rose gently
and carried us away
    in summer sleep.

Norman Elder

Love-in-a-Mist

I met my love in a mist down in the meadow,
The water-meadow, winter-stiff and bare;
    Over the frozen fen her apparition,
A breathing shadow seen in middle air.

Cold frosted twigs unseen brushed on our shoulders,
Tall trees loomed out beyond our firmament:
    Hid in our ghostly ring from all beholders
No watching eye shall spy the way we went.

Close side to side, the world dissolves in whiteness,
We two alone, bewildered, jubilant;
    No touch, no sound, no human exultation.
In that cold circle is our covenant.

Fiona Kidman

The Blue Dress

There was me
getting off the little plane
from the north
and careless
enough with my hair
undone and wearing
jeans as if
I was one of the film moguls
riding in the little plane
with me

and then there was you
there was you love
waiting in the hum and buzz
waiting in the big terminal
in the strange city

amongst the false gods
waiting there for me
as well, only I didn't hear
them or the calls
on the speakers in the big space
because it was you love
yes you alone and brave and out

        on your own
at last:
   hungry of course
and smaller
than I thought
in a spreading blue
denim maternity dress with frills
at the neck straightening
me up so I'd pass well enough
to be with you and neither
of us hearing the voices
calling me, because
I was
with you love I was
with you
in your glowing growing blue dress.

Ian Wedde

It's Time

A beautiful evening, early summer.
I'm walking from the hospital. His head
was a bright nebula

　　　　　　　a firmament
swimming in the vulva's lens . . . *the colour
of stars*/ 'Terraces the colour of stars . . .'

I gazed through my tears.

　　　　　　　The gifts of the dead
crown the heads of the newborn　　　　　She said
'It's time' & now I have a son　　　　　time for

naming the given
　　　　　　　the camellia
which is casting this hoar of petals (stars?)
on the grass . . . all winter the wind kept from
the south, driving eyes & heart to shelter.
Then came morning when she said 'It's time, it's
time!' time's
　　　　　　　careless nebula of blossom/

Hone Tuwhare

Lovers

(On the occasion of a visit to New Zealand by Germaine Greer)

In a packed house we pressed
into a knee-high row
of seats. It was hot.

The chairman began again
when we were quite settled.
I sniffed. Fastidiously.

Indifferent, you blamed me
for using all the hot water.
Then, you should have
showered with me, I muttered.

It's a you-and-me smell, you
said with deliberation,
breast heavy-loll against me.

Arms lowly, and beseeching
heaven, I juggled my eye-balls;
your lizard-eyes fixed wise
on me.

The speaker was a woman who spoke
plainly, but only one plain
word I caught from her all
evening. I think she said fuck:

and O,
said everyone turning to look
at us.

Brian Turner

Shining

Standing on the dark wet road watching
the grass waving
the leaves on the trees
the light on the harbour
your eyes   the sky
the few hesitant white clouds
all are shining

and the black hides
and lustrous eyes
of the cows
they too are shining
as they rock
slowly
downhill
and turn and stand
motionless

our hands touch briefly
and all there is to it
is there in your eyes
bravely
shining

Mohammad Amir

Love

Two lovers
Sitting at the coast of a lake
In the light of moon
Talking about their romance

Oh moon:
Don't think that you're the only one
Which has the sweet and bright light
Be aware:
My beloved's face
Is brighter than you

He is my tears
He always lives in my wet eyes
What a strange person:
Lives in the house of water

How long we'll hide our love
One day
we should tell the world
The tale of our unique romance

Don't go so early
Night's still travelling

Keep the voice down
the silence of night
listens to us

Iain Sharp

The Plan

Heart of my heart
I've put hours of thought into this
and tonight when we meet
I want to kiss

neglected parts of you
like your elbows and eyelids
the peaks of your ankles
the backs of your knees.

Is this asking too much?
The night sky is so vast
and both sides of my family
tend to die young.

Cilla McQueen

Crikey

I can't think straight
my words spin off
in sugar and spice
god you're nice
I've got a running filmstrip in my head of you
every time I close my eyes
I close my eyes quite often
I feel so good
I feel like a morning
a kiss on a ferris wheel
in a tunnel of love
I'm not quite sure what's happening
but your image is in me like a scent
all the roses in the garden are opening up at once
it's raining big round drops
of extraordinary sweetness
let me be serious
I'm in love with you
                  I think of you
at every
        turn   move
my hand
        your eyes   your hand
(crikey)
do the washing
dream on the doorstep
clean all the windows at high speed
get lost
stare into space
                watch a
green caterpillar

spinning enough
amazingly fine silk
to let itself down smoothly
from the very top
leaf
of the tree.

A.R.D. Fairburn

Winter Night

The candles gutter and burn out,
  and warm and snug we take our ease,
and faintly comes the wind's great shout
  as he assails the frozen trees.

The vague walls of this little room
  contract and close upon the soul;
deep silence hangs amid the gloom;
  no sound but the small voice of the coal.

Here in this sheltered firelit place
  we know not wind nor shivering tree;
we two alone inhabit space,
  locked in our small infinity.

This is our world, where love enfolds
  all images of joy, all strife
resolves in peace: this moment holds
  within its span the sum of life.

For Time's ghost: these reddening coals
  were forest once ere he'd begun,
and now from dark and timeless boles
  we take the harvest of the sun;

and still the flower-lit solitudes
  are radiant with the springs he stole
where violets in those buried woods
  wake little blue flames in the coal.

Great stars may shine above this thatch;
  beyond these walls perchance are men
with laws and dreams: but our thin latch
  holds all such things beyond our ken.

The fire that lights our cloudy walls
   now fails beneath the singing pot,
and as the last flame leaps and falls
   the far wall is and then is not.

Now lovelier than firelight is the gleam
   of dying embers, and your face
shines through the pathways of my dream
   like young leaves in a forest place.

Mary Stanley

Per Diem et per Noctem

Birds in their oratory of leaves
Clamour at morning over my love.
All waters praise him, the sea harbours
from harm, all islands are his neighbour
and rain at daybreak feathers his peace
softer than pillows or my kiss.

O may his lucky hand at noon
pluck down the sun, all day his keen
eye be darkened by no cloud.
Sky-walker, the lonely hawk, applaud
his purpose, the equipoise among
cliff and rock, his difficult song.

O never may night confound or send
him lost into that hinterland
far from my coasts. Where is your moon,
Endymion, trimming her thin
flame to light my love? The world
lifts its shoulder to shelter him curled
in the lap of sleep. By falling star
I wish all his tomorrows fair.

Meg Campbell

After Loving

While we lie hidden in ourselves
a moment longer, two colours
light up a world within.
At first, Chinese red
because we are happy,
and then emerald,
the god-green of peace
that follows when you follow me
while my hands
wing their separate flights
along your gullies.

Hone Tuwhare

Yes

I like the Way
you slip out
of your things
pausing
between zip and
catch of breath
as if you were
punctuating
a movement: a phrase
of love. God

it cheers me
when you move with
purpose: animal
grace and awareness
of the urgency with
which agents
of locomotion take
us from a to z
table to bed and
back to the floor
again: hip hip

Yes: and I love
the way our limbs
construct
a superstructure
to a heavenly
accommodation: cheers

me no end

Dinah Hawken

1 (Meeting on the Tideline)

At last we're in each other's arms.
The dark one and the fair one.

I've been waiting for you
for so long.

I'd forgotten you.
I'd forgotten who you are.

This is me, she says,
stepping back and standing
like Christ with her palms to the front
showing where her heart is.

But there are no wounds.
Not a trace of them. No thorns.
No halo. Just her, with no embellishments.

Vivienne Plumb

Before the Operation

You'll be there in white
you'll drop into the bottom of nowhere
when they give you the needle
I'll hold your hand
while you flake out.

Forefinger and thumb
we're that close,
moi et vous,
(or rather *tu*),
sometimes so hair's breadth
we can't breathe.

The body has a terrestrial
magnetism even when it's unconscious
but the soul
is the one to watch,
possessing wings of its own,
I'll have to weight yours
telling you the wonderful things
about you, yourself, and your life.

J.R. Hervey

Even So Came Love

Treading unknown ways and lovely beyond
All lonely dreams, 'tis Love herself I see—
'Tis Love herself who pledges sanctuary
In bosom quiet as a twilight pond.

Out of the unguessed deep the song is blown,
And all earth's voices die. What shall compare
With that by which all other things are fair,
Who shall contend with Love's unravaged throne?

As comes the moon into surrendered skies,
Even so came Love to whom I yield me now,
Deliberate hand and heart and dreaming brow.
And song-sweet lips and beauty-haunted eyes.

J.C. Sturm

Before Dawn, Before Dark

For Peter

Do not go with the dark,
Lie with me a little longer
Skin to skin,
My hands resting here
In the valley of your shoulders.

Take my mouth with your mouth,
Breathe my breath
As your own,
With passion protesting
Surely now we are as one

Until a wintry-eyed sun
Stands up and stares you down.

> Do not leave with the light,
> Walk with me a little while
> Side by side,
> My heart resting here
> In the haven of your hand.

> Match my thoughts with your thoughts,
> Ease my hurt
> As your own,
> With tenderness caring
> To make us truly one

> Until our short day is ended
> And the long night begun.

Laura Ranger

Mum

Her hair curls
like fern fronds.

Her eyes are like
speckled green birds' eggs.

Her glasses are two pools
of clear water.

Her nose is blunt.

Her hands are wrinkled and kind.
She reaches out to touch me.

I love my mum
forty four million
times around the world.

James K. Baxter

My Love Late Walking

My love late walking in the rain's white aisles
I break words for, though many tongues
Of night deride and the moon's boneyard smile

Cuts to the quick our newborn sprig of song.
See and believe, my love, the late yield
Of bright grain, the sparks of harvest wrung

From difficult joy. My heart is an open field.
There you may stray wide or stand at home
Nor dread the giant's bone and broken shield

Or any tendril locked on a thunder stone,
Nor fear, in the forked grain, my hawk who flies
Down to your feathered sleep alone

Striding blood coloured on a wind of sighs.
Let him at the heart of your true dream move,
My love, in the lairs of hope behind your eyes.

I sing, to the rain's harp, of light renewed,
The black tares broken, fresh the phoenix light
I lost among time's rags and burning tombs.

My love walks long in harvest aisles tonight.

Alan Riach

That Silence

I kept thinking of that silence we fell into,
sometime after the shower, it seemed the last,
when every touch was wanting more, denied
and every time we held
                    each other, we held on
time; and of, when I held you then, so
close, looking over your shoulder, as we were
dressed and standing by your suitcase by the door
looking back on that great broad bed,
its white sheets tumbled, broken into Alps—
and I've been thinking too about the way, then,
we moved away so quick,
                    and the way
I could say nothing; and neither could you—

that silence that we let ourselves fall into—

so that now, we can break it again.

Bill Manhire

Love Poem

There is no question
of choice, but it takes
a long time.

Love's vacancies, the eye
& cavity, track
back to embraces

where the spine bends
& quietens
like smoke in the earth.

Your tongue, touching on song,
darkens all songs. Your touch
is almost a signature.

Kendrick Smithyman

Kingfisher Song

A yellow-breasted bird
heraldic upon a rock
devised himself to give back
due light to the afternoon.
Who from his posing took
strength, as from the sun?

I gave all my strength to a woman
and she returned it each day
miraculously; who could play
a right music for my ear,
in the deep of her body could cry
that my inmost bone should hear.

When winter rode on the wind
she walked the rain out and threw
gay mischiefs on a low
most sobersided stream,
and on that kingfisher who
sat shrugged in his harmless dream.

Keith Sinclair

To Her for Christmas

dancing you are my festival,
yet in your arms my seasons
are at rest, and never peace
lay deeper on the seas, while I
your shepherd, watch the flock
of hopes we keep for newer summers,
count them on your hair and
in your lips and touched
my blood goes carolling
down all the hills you farmed in me
and celebrates your breath.
it is no blasphemy since I must say
that all my nights are holier
because you bring the air
of older customs to my ways
and make each day a new nativity.

Lauris Edmond

Doubletake

I saw without looking flamingos were flying,
pohutukawas doing cartwheels over the hill,
the garden full of gazelles, dancing for sure . . .

then it was daylight, morning; Thursday;
your pillow slightly dented, spectacles left
by the bed, your special smell. I looked out,

saw a crimson launch stooging over the harbour,
two starlings in the pine tree, an orange arctotis
in bloom by the path—but everything queerly bright,

so I stared in disbelief. And I suddenly thought,
gazelles, etc., are OK: this is love's greater
invention, that it can take a red boat,

gossipy birds, an ancient familiar daisy, and
remake them, leaving all things their familiarity,
giving each a surpassing strangeness.

Alistair Te Ariki Campbell

Bon Voyage

to Meg

Crossing the straits is easy
As sleeping with you, my sweet:
The waves just keep slipping away
Like the bedclothes from our feet.

A salt moon leans to the mast,
White as your head on my arm—
I'm afraid of the lights on the sea,
I'm afraid of the calm.

A gull falls away in the dark,
Like your lost hand under a sheet
When hunger is deep as the ocean
And there's no advance or retreat.

Drowning is easy, my darling,
As when foundering lip to lip
Horizons topple and vanish
And into your breathing I slip.

Cilla McQueen

Wham Bananaskin Catapult

just when you're least expecting it
you think you've got it right at last
then wham bananaskin catapult
two make love in
softness & symmetry
hardness & nectar
shake twist tumble kiss fracture
falling in love oh no this is impossible

barriers have been set up
roadblocks & heavy artillery
nobody is getting through
nothing at all is getting through
& then you
kiss me crack my shell crack my island
crack my heart
& fill me up with
clean & unpredictable
smoothness & touching our
hands over each other
jesus I can hardly think about it
it's gonna drive me crazy oh no
love shake sex twist
this is extremely serious
this is falling in love
falling in love oh no this is impossible

Hone Tuwhare

When the Karaka Trees Whistled and Said to Us:
Kia Kaha!

Sallyann took my hand
        as we walked deeper into the bush: the moon, care-
fully parting the leaves of the Karaka trees—got a better peek
        at us, surely.

Between Sallyann's thighs I kneeled. With my deft tongue
        I parted her bush neatly up the centre
                                when o,
                        God was there
                    wet-nosed, n'all—

a belligerent guardian—whom I soon licked into an understanding
and shape; an upstanding sentry now guarding the outermost and the
                        innermost parts of Sallyann's
                        moistened lips—
        the holy-templed arch-way of her—her offertory box
                    unburgled and she yielding
                        at last to my surly
                    hurly-burly, come-in-early
                            and

ooof, she said
(to my aaahs)
and

aaah, she said
(to my ooofs)
and

do you know, the piratical bloody trees
were mimic-ing our sighs,
our cries A N D gingering-up commonplace crudities
with raucous hey-nonny NOES and a yo-ho hoe-ing'n all
that carry-on—
but mostly
we were oblivious to them all—
oblivious even to the crisp dead leaves beneath us
crackling and cracking up at the way
Sallyann and I were doing it OUR way
but in our own smug warm togetherness
we thanked us (God, n'all) for everything
with the moon, like a one-eyed owl not
showing any respect but grinning hugely n'all:
hugely.

Bob Orr

Love Poem

In your eyes
there is a balcony

In my heart
there is a hammock

Let's lie
there
& watch those birds
that fly

With wings
like hospital beds
& hope
that they make it into heaven.

John Barr

Meet Me When the Moon is Up

Meet me when the moon is up
    And blinkin' ower the brae,
O meet me by the trystin' tree,
    My own sweet lovely May;
There I will be awaitin' thee;
    When shadows speil the hill:
When, minglin' with the balmy breeze,
    Come echoes of the rill.

O meet me in the bushy dell,
    Thou darling of my heart!
Why should we meet, and meet so oft,
    And yet so often part?
With hope deferred the heart turns sad,
    O haste that happy day,
When I may ca' ye a' my ain,
    My own sweet lovely May!

I ken your father frowns on me,
    Because that I am poor;
Your mother thwarts my fervent love,
    Wi' a' a mother's power;
But love was never bought with gold,
    Whatever men may say;
For love is wealth in humble ha',
    My own sweet lovely May!

They've met beside the trystin' tree,
    The moments quickly flew;
He clasped her to his beatin' heart,
    His May was kind and true:
She's gi'en her heart, she's gi'en her han',
    His wedded wife to be;
My blessing on their virtuous love,
    And on the trystin' tree.

J.R. Hervey

She was My Love Who Could Deliver

She was my love who could deliver
From paws of pain and melancholy,
And light the lamps that burn forever,
And cleanse a page of screeds of folly,
And with a motion of her hand
Could reap a harvest on my land.

And she could melt an iron mood,
And lashing chords with love were softer,
And she could bring my course to good,
Could renovate with raining laughter,
And eye and heart her beauty brace
When death approached with peering face.

Against a secret shaft of malice
Piercing my solitary isle
She would defend with flying solace,
And visitations of her smile,
And from the spirit's blank occasions,
And from the craft of days and seasons
She was my love who could deliver.

J.C. Sturm

Maori to Pakeha

for Peter

You there
I mean you
Beak-nosed hairy-limbed narrow-footed
Pakeha you
Milton directing your head
Donne pumping your heart
You singing
Some old English folksong
Meanwhile trampling Persia
Or is it India, underfoot
With such careless feet.

Where do you think you're going?
You must be colour-blind.
Can't you see you've strayed
Into another colour zone?
This is brown country, man
Brown on the inside
As well as the outside
Brown through and through
Even the music is brown
Like us.

So what are you after?
All the land has long gone
With the tupuna.
Nothing left to colonise now
Except the people.
Do you plan to play
Antony to my Cleopatra?
I mean
Who do you think you are?

Tell me all I want to know
Before you crook that finger again
Smile me another crooked smile.
Give your mihi tonight
Korero mai
Till dawn breaks with a waiata
Meanwhile holding me gently
Firmly captive
Here, in the tight curve
Of your alien arm
My dear

Oh my dear.

Kathleen Grattan

A Sudden Radiance

It rained all night
the lancewood hung its leaves

and raindrops shivered.

A winter sun slid clever fingers
through the fern

flicked on the power

and every glistening leaf
gleamed copper.

Then I recalled

your sudden radiance
when I touched you.

Bernadette Hall

Lovesong

for John

missing you
like I've been hit
and missing you
for years

in a doorway
somewhere between
the kitchen
and the laundry

missing the way
you tell me every day
I'm beautiful

putting a kiss
on my forehead
when I'm sick

and on my tongue
a sweet exotic tincture
with your tongue

we could call it
ha-ka-ta-ra-mea

Allen Curnow

A Woman in Mind

i

I have lit a single lamp
and laid my fire beneath
for cold faint-sun days
of frost and cloudy breath.

Her eyes my early lamp
in this winter of the heart;
her body, limbs burning,
holds bitterness apart.

Shadows prank my walls;
outside, rain is flying:
ere my light and my fire die
I too shall be dying.

ii

Your face between my hands
and your eyes open to me,
it is as if I stood
beside a great sea;
for nothing is so still
or perfect in its pride
or such deep semblance, as
the flesh I stand beside.

iii

My hands worship
you with suppliant touch
in whatever part seeking
to know you bodily.

Nothing is withheld
from us in our free
city of love, we conceal
not from any sense.

To shrink from flesh
is to offend the spirit—
who can divide them
one from the other?

Now you receive
hand at breast and thigh,
I suppliant; but soon
equal communion.

iv

As the green music compassing
all earth that listens in the spring
so is the semblance when your nearness
shakes taut and void to broken clearness
and music, music cries to be
about the way you walk to me.

v

Who am I
that I should own
so fair a field
and meet, for yield?

That in this earth's
deep, sweet warmth
my seed should stir
(the sun loves her)

drinking bright rain
in womb of tenderness,
god's gate, the same,
Mary without blame?

Since it is mine
this earth, her flesh,
bears that which I
wanting, should die.

vi

By pain outspoken
a precious thing is broken,
peace destroyed by pain
no words can bring again.

May sun never bless me
and loud winds oppress me
if from me is heard
a destructive word.

Shut my mouth upon your breast;
now I have confessed,
on my lips let move
breath only of love.

vii

In the time of your conceiving
which shall be in spring
we shall die with flowers, together
in all our blossoming.

A rose shall ask your lips
close, as never before
when summer has deepened
and life is at the door.

Autumn shall bring us then
leaves' grace in falling,
wind-lightened, lost suns
without pain recalling.

Winter, not an enemy
to earth's true lover,
but womb of new sowing,
shall cover us over.

R.A.K. Mason

Flow at Full Moon

Your spirit flows out over all the land between
    your spirit flows out as gentle and limpid as milk
    flows on down ridge and through valley as soft and serene
    as the light of the moon that sifts down through its light sieve of silk

The long fingers of the flow press forward, the whole hand follows
    easily the fingers creep they're your hair's strands that curl
    along the land's brow, your hair dark-bright gleaming on heights and
        hollows
    and the moon illumines the flow with mother of pearl

Beloved your love is poured to enchant all the land
    the great bull falls still the opossum turns from his chatter
    and the thin nervous cats pause and the strong oak-trees stand
    entranced and the gum's restless bark-strip is stilled from its clatter

Your spirit flows out from your deep and radiant nipples
    and the whole earth turns tributary all her exhalations
    wave up in white breath and are absorbed in the ripples
    that pulse like a bell along the blood from your body's pulsations

And as the flow settles down to the sea it nets me about
    with a noose of one soft arm stretched out from its course:
    oh loved one my dreams turn from sleep: I shall rise and go out
    and float my body into the flow and press back till I find its source.

K.O. Arvidson

By the Clear Fountain

A long time you've had all my love,
And I shall love forever.

So fresh and cool the falling rain
this fountain in the white sun makes,
it seems the very water holds
your dearest self within its folds
of shining cloth that combs and breaks
unchangingly, while I complain.

For I should love you more, to see
how fair a face that cloth conceals.
My thoughts you lead unseen to sights
impossible by known delights
to gauge or more than guess how feels
completely this desire in me.

Yet if I give you hands and face,
that might disturb the fountain's flow.
In water-lace and rose I dress
the echo of this tenderness,
another love, a girl I know
as fresh as rain, with rain's white grace.

The flower I place among her hair
is fountain-like, as she herself is.
Changing, it blooms and overflows,
yet still remains essential rose,
like water where you dwell, because
you flower in rise and changing there.

Peter Bland

Bear Dance

For Beryl

To bring you to my bed
I must dramatize myself:
I must walk through the house
in primary colours.

How else can I be seen
among all the children and flowers
among all the music and mirrors
among all the open windows
that surround you?

I have to shout
to wear bright shirts
to dance up and down
rattling the cups in the kitchen.

The children laugh
They say I'm a bear.
They like it best when I roll on the ground.
They say there's a dancing bear in the house.

But this is my love dance.
Aheee . . . I bellow . . .
clicking my throat like the starlings
in the early morning
when they think they've swallowed the sun.

This, I say, is my love dance.
Later I shall paint your image.
There'll be a bold but awkward tenderness

trembling in each line . . .
I'll be struggling to overcome my clumsiness
with the strength of my love.

These are my charms—
my bear dance and my image of you.
With these I'll bring you to my bed
again and again.

When you see me in my bright shirt
when you hear neighbours and friends complaining
saying I'm loud and heavy-footed
remember that my dance is for you.
It's in your sole honour.
It has to compete with your silence
and with the other silences that go on and on
like the sky through this open window
for ever . . .

Denis Glover

In Needless Doubt

Blow hot the wind, blow cold.
Soon we will both be old,
Wormed with regrets.

Oh let's take
Time's whiskers with a tug,
Light up and let time lag.

Brightness

I am bright with the wonder of you
And the faint perfume of your hair

I am bright with the wonder of you
You being far away or near

I am bright with the wonder of you
Warmed by your eyes' blue fire

I am bright with the wonder of you
and your mind's open store

Peggy Dunstan

Even in Sleep

Even in sleep,
moon lubricated
locked in love our limbs tangle,
silvered by sweat
            and light
they shine
in the night's spangle.
            Softly
the sea breathes
over the sands and shingle
            softly
you move against me
and our dreams mingle.
Even in sleep
your voice calls
light as wind in the poplar tree
curving through leaves
            of gold
and when you enter me
            you are the horned moon
you are the stars
the sun.
You are the flame, all things.
The song ended
            and the song begun.

Michael Harlow

from *Poem Then, for Love*

2

And just now

The way light swarms over
your shoulders.
The day is remarkable that lifts
the town to walk on stilts.
The sun wheels down,
windows shine.

In the crowns of flowers
small fires leap; seeds spill
in the bright air.
Like planets spinning
into sight, passatempo our bodies
turn the hours.

For love your hair sings,
and earth's curve.
For love I pour light
into your body like this—
oh, there is music to be heard,
and just now.

Bub Bridger

Love Poem

Yesterday
I watched you walk
Slim and neat-footed
Through the Sunday Market
Your bright clothes glowed
Golden as the leaves
At your feet and your hair

Was on fire you were happy
And happiness shines on you
Like the sun on daisies
—you lose that wariness
The watchful knowledge
Of pain

Suzy!
My first born
My April child
Wearing Autumn like a silk dress
Beautiful
At the Sunday Market

Keith Sinclair

The Lovers

She has a bellbird in her breast—
O bird go singing down my throat—
And in the flametree of desire
She builds her hot and honeyed nest.

Those lips are red but never say
What burns in her bright hibiscus veins.
I ask, what keeps her sad and still?
She says, 'my love', and dark goes day.

O heart be nimble, pulse with hers,
She may not speak that word again.
Swoop with her mood from breath to breath,
From sleet to summer, kiss to curse.

O rare and desired, desiring pair,
Twin parakeets, feathered with tropical fire,
Tracing your parallels in the air
To meet in an infinite everywhere.

Anton Vogt

Marriage

Girl: If you will give your hand
I'll give my heart;
For vows go lightly where life's short but sweet,
And youth gives youth its answer—understand?
There'll be no kissing when we are apart
And in the land you leave for we'll not meet.

Soldier: Then come, I'll give myself as lightly,
Yielding more gladly than to harsher steel;
Shelving the morrow's menace, I shall bless
A love that does not burn less brightly
Because its hungry flames reveal
Our mutual loneliness.

The Wind: Here then, while earth and heaven sunder
The age-old bonds of decency and love,
Let these two come together if they must;
While warring continents like ships go under
Their temporary love redeems
The actions of the just.

Jenny Bornholdt

The Loved One

Ah   you
the loved one
coming down out of the sky
like rain   your arms wide
branches   your narrowness
a song for the strong ones
a line coming across
the room to greet me.
Your hands find me out
in the world   my arms
I will take you in till
the morning and a sky

sharp with the sounds
of birds. For all of this
we take to the water
chance on an island small
as a raisin   love,
this is surprise
this is our very own
continent.

Jan Kemp

Poem

It was your face.
It was shy.
We walked.
It was your head.
It was lit with sun.
I unbuckled your belt.
Hush, don't speak,
the yellow flowers are bursting.

Poem

A puriri moth's wing
lies light in my hand—

my breath can lift it

light as this torn wing
we lie on love's breath.

Ian Wedde

Drought

A woman in love's
abstracted, her mouth turns
down at the corners,
the world presses in on her,
at night in the room where she lies
the planets enter!   so close it all is
but she cannot touch it.

All day the sound of that distance,
all night the sound

which her heart measures.
Where is the beginning of it?
Where is the end?
She can start anywhere

& any time.
But she cannot

oh start at all.

Erick Brenstrum

First Love

I

your image
before me like a flag
fills with the wind
a bright cloud after dawn
that folds into
the blue spaces of memory

II

your back like a harp
my hands melt with the strings
music enters my arms
the bones hum

III

your smile
a gift like the sun
I take to the streets to find it

Basil Dowling

The Best of All

Sing love the secret balm the mother bears
For pains and panics of our infant years.

Sing love the child, and love the morning time
When sense and spirit peal a perfect chime.

Sing love the wisdom unto fullness come
That calls men brothers and the world a home.

Sing love the purpose passionate and true
To build for beauty and make all things new.

Sing love the trumpet, torch, and golden thread
Reaching the distant, bringing back the dead.

Sing love the heavenward way since life began,
The Christmas and the Christ in every man.

K.O. Arvidson

Riding the Pendulum

Your bruises appal me.
There is no rhetoric equal to them,
their dark shining, the savage
trace of passion's colour within their night.
They're all my making, and I'd
salve them, I would
substitute these for them:
your body's own light, all
obedience, birthday's white
communion.
          The moon to your feet
I'd have you in, and your crowning face
an angel, a fond renaissance,
hopefully, not with prophetic burials
scarred, or torn
with the vanishing of these hands, but
borne aloft, above thin whips whimpering
home, and their fall of snow.
Small cries of you are an island,
riding the pendulum. Why do you
sway so to my tidal risings? Why
does diminishing pain I bind you with
assault like kindness!
Morning and night I am the wine
that only you believe,
the gall and vinegar.
The chains.
I am the blood that darkens in your veins.

Ian Wedde

Beautiful Golden Girl of the Sixties

Beautiful
golden girl of the Sixties
I remember your mouth
under the Pacific stars

I remember your delicate pale breast
in some dark old car backseat
the salt beachparty flavour of you in sandy tussock

I remember you stumble-drunk in an alley
& made clumsy by desire
in your very best dress

& the sound of summer after-work traffic on the hill
where you shared my narrow bed
when the night-scented datura lilies
began to breathe into the room
your thighs pale as lilies
their evening nectar

& how could you forget when
we managed it in the toilet
of the old clang-bang all-night Limited from Wellington
to Auckland, must've been dead of night
near frosty Taumaranui

oh ho beautiful golden girl of the Sixties

or the time at dawn in a narrow bunk
on the all-night ferryboat from Christchurch
to Wellington, & the tealady
never spilt a drop

Once on the top platform
of a slide in the children's playground
at birdsong dusk in Coromandel
in summer & someone nearby yelled out
'There's a time & place for everything!'
—quite right! And

I remember the elevator
of the hotel St George in Beirut
both of us crazy from separation at gunpoint
& that night parked in fresh pinegroves
above the city, a patrol with torches & machineguns
& us stark naked & covered with blood
from your nose that I'd knocked in fright
& I couldn't find my glasses

obvious we weren't spies
we were just investigating each other

hey beautiful golden girl of the Sixties

something we did also in hotpools & in cool rivers
& in baths & in showers & in the sea

in grass (often)
up in a tree (pohutukawa)
in sand

on floors, carpets, chairs, tables
in kitchens, dining rooms, living-rooms, lounges,
bathrooms
and in very many bedrooms

filled with woodsmoke & mosquitoes & the sound
of the sea or the sound
of city traffic or of wind, or opening wide windows
to the stars, the clouds

and in tents & Kombis &
hotel & motel rooms & in cheap spermy motorcamps
with the smells of last summer's crayfish dinner
round the cookhouse, piddle under the pines

oh oh beautiful golden girl of the Sixties

poor blanket student cot, green nikau palm arbour
car backseat, cool heaven of wide whitesheeted bed
Sri-Lankan resthouse, sexy Swiss featherbed
Tunisian bandit pinewood, dim cheap Damascus hotel
sad dark South London, sodden sheets in Denpasar
Otago winter quilts

maybe mostly the wide cool beds
where we lay heads together
talking when it was quiet

straight, drunk, stoned, stopped, speeding, tripped
sad, happy, tired, daytime, night, morning, hot, cold
fucking & tasting, your huge flavours & groan
our hands & mouths, your bubble saliva, my come
weary & gay, your smell, the bitter fuck of rage
in silence, with laughter, to music, meanwhile-conversation
'that was great'—'that was terrible'—'again'—'later'—
your tongue, your eyes, your frightening tears
your giggle, your toughness, your smile
your shudder, your sardonic forbearing, your sudden sweat
your stoopid, your brave terror, your

your body where I dip my chipped cup
like a despairing pilgrim

ah 'my' beautiful golden girl of the Sixties

mother of my sons, your tired
lovely body where I bring my terminal need
where I stoop with cracked shaking lips

beatup puppydog cock, sad smile
& pounding heart, saying Show me again
this everyday miracle
how you bring forth such floods of seed from a fool

Jenny Bornholdt

Lake Rotoiti

Grey herons
delicate
on the lawn

swans tipped
up, their red beaks
grazing weed.

Quickly, quickly
the grey rain comes
across the lake

then later, water
dark
under the black
hillside.

In the evenings
we listen for
the pianist's
breath, the click
of a cuff button against
the saxophone.

Night was meant
for this
the taking of
one body into
another, the dark
cry.

Then, suddenly, the
body of morning
coming through
the door.

We'll take
the dinghy out
to the yellow buoy,
moor there, slip into
the dark lake
unsure of what's below but
chance it anyway, whatever
it is.

Part 2

A straight account is difficult

Meg Campbell

This Morning at Dawn

Pirate! I woke this morning
to find you anchored in me.
You had come in through the Heads
at first light. My plump whiteness
amuses you vastly. Your teeth gleam
and your eyes are dark slits.
Shamelessly you have beached
your long-boat high on the sand . . .

You handsome bastard,
how is it that you are
so very sure of your ground?
The tide is going out, amigo—
take care that the water
doesn't drown you, leaving only
your cocked hat floating
on the surface . . . Is it true, then,
that pirates never learn to swim?

from *A Diary 79*

How can we (seriously)
separate when you
are as rash as a scattering
of stars, and as loopy
as a rainbow with its ends tied?

How can I impress on you
my doubts, while we sit
in a mud-splattered V Dub
with my red felt hat
squashed in the back?

Brent Southgate

Windfalls

Love, we arrange ourselves too much,
like awkward flowers in vases:
let's be more accidental to each other.

Something might grow from that. Just any-old-how,
like marigolds that strollers and lovers chance on
in what used to be gardens;

sooty-gold and surprised through the rubbish,
and against odds, they bloom from a soil
secret, disregarded, sweetened by windfalls.

The Disappearance

Lounging now in the warm smell of cushions
after that sunlit bread and salad and wine,
my head is a sort of jug the sun has emptied
and the flies think I am part of the furniture.
I shade my eyes, and float into
a slow-motion novel of nineteen ten
in which you figure as a domestic poetry.
It occurs to me: if I sit very still,
I will be totally happy.

But it goes. It goes on, and
more and more, nothing begins to be said.
I watch the hair swing shut over your face
as you sit darning socks to the music
of Mozart's last illness.
Already we disappear to each other.

Brent Southgate

Tactics

That day, your talk was so anywhere and quick
you were a fantail in a schoolroom, playing
in a sunlight high away from me.

In the end, lost, I held out both hands
and made kissing sounds with my lips,
calling you down.

Ian Wedde

Homecoming

That's all you know, gifted with love.
Your back view fills me with tenderness,
remorse, passion that needs to move slowly,
postponing its ambitions. Why
remorse? Be honest, you have a hard
time of it, Beloved, rose of all the world,
back turned to me. In thought
I reach round you, your breast warms
my fingers, I send one hand down your belly.
November misty evening, the bridges
arch their spines in fading light.
Slow pulse of evening, the slow river, certain
& patient, passing into their next days.
Your hair has grown longer, to your shoulders.
When we get back you can cut
it & feel the warm breeze on your nape.

Robin Hyde

Silence

I am tired of all voices. Friend and fool
Have come too nearly with me to the shrine
That is the secret kept by wind and pine.
Now, when the shadowy hands of dusk are cool
About my eyes, shall silence like a god
Drive them with whips of starlight from his stairs.
Only the small grass striving in its clod,
Only the stream, that fragile moonlight bears
Like blossoms on its breast, move in this place,

All earth lies still as some beloved face
Whose dreaming mouth and deep-curved eyelids make
Bridges to God that lightest sound would break,
Towers where one word would seem iconoclast . . .
Yet if through darkening trees you came at last,
Wearing the dew of meadows on your shoon,
And in your eyes the blessing of the moon,
I think it would be well. I think our greeting
Would be as quiet as two rivers meeting,
Which, drawn together, sparkling up in foam,
Slide into one bright seeking; and our home
Should be the furthest longing of pale seas,
Beyond the purple caverns of the trees.

Fiona Farrell

Love Songs

Seven Wishes

A straight account is difficult
so let me define seven wishes:

that you should fit inside me neat as the stuffing in an olive
that you should stand inside the safe circle of my eye
that you should sing, clear, on the high rock of my skull
that you should swing wide on the rope of my hair
that you should cross rivers of blood, mountains of bone
that I should touch your skin through the hole in your tee shirt
that we should exchange ordinary tales.

Full

Today I am full to the brim with you.
You lip about my edges clear as rain.
When I'm not looking you spill
onto lists and books and what
to have for dinner.
I catch the round drop of you
full on my finger.

The day tastes entirely of you.

I lick this good day.

Spring

That duck racing for the reeds
on wheeled feet and after her a
drake penis grabbing a plastic
hose inches of it zoom into the
reeds and all that rough spring
stuff. Tulips in mincing rows
fart scarlet cats nest under
the Civic Centre and pop
kittens like black peas and you
strip your white winter body and
paint the bedroom lickety lick
madonna blue because nothing's
sacred and everything's blessed.

Bill Manhire

Poem

When we touch,
forests enter our bodies.

The dark wind shakes the branch.
The dark branch shakes the wind.

The Proof

She did not speak to me yesterday
All day there was silence
By this I was hurt
I walked down the street
Unable to think of anything
But her: that is how these things
Affect you
              today she says
Good morning, kisses me
So I am sullen, I do not reply
I think I must love her

The Elaboration

There was a way out of here:
it went off in the night
licking its lips.

The door flaps like a great wing:
I make fists at the air
and long to weaken.

Ah, to visit you
is the plain thing,
and I shall not come to it.

John Allison

In/Fidelities

1

when he went out
she said nothing to him

when he returned
she didn't turn away

when he explained
there wasn't any anger
in her quiet reply

instead she looked
at him as though
there never had been
much between them

2

she watches the gulls
wheeling over the sea

he watches the girls
sunbathing on the beach

when he looks at her
he sees someone
he's never known

when she looks at him
she sees him

Hone Tuwhare

You Have to Come First Before You Can Go

Oh it's true—it's true. And it gets harder at
    night, thinking of you. Harder still appease
    an appetite more constantly in bud with your
    comings rather than your goings. For it has
    no useful name except, love; seemingly
    old-fashioned, and imprecise.

And if the sky were unpeopled—the stars and planets
    have a falling out with it—it would make
    a memorable mark; like my nail-gouged buttocks
    that you've tinctured pink, the shattered bed
    frame—mute evidence that we'd got into it.
    You'll just have to cut your nails, or wear
    boxing gloves, and may I say, in a reserved
    judgment, that our exulting most moving parts
    are compatible?

And you, you
    at the most extreme sou'westerly end now
    of spun kilometres—to whom phone calls dialled
    around midnight might assuage—in return
    call down on me a good night; a dark warm coat
    to nudge into and hug.

C.K. Stead

from *Quesada*

'Je pense . . . aux vaincus!'

1

All over the plain of the world lovers are being hurt.
The spring wind takes up their cries and scatters them to the clouds.
Juan Quesada hears them. By the world at large they go unheard.
Only those in pain can hear the chorus of pain.
High in the air over winds that shake the leaves
High over traffic, beyond bird call, out of the reach of silence
These lovers are crying out because the spring has hurt them.
No one dies of that pain, some swear by it, a few will live with it always,
No one mistakes it for the lamentations of hell
Because there is a kind of exaltation in it
More eloquent than the tongues of wind and water
More truthful than the sibylline language of the leaves
The cry of the injured whose wounds are dear to them
The howl of the vanquished who cherish their defeat.

Fleur Adcock

Double-Take

You see your next-door neighbour from above,
from an upstairs window, and he reminds you
of your ex-lover, who is bald on top,
which you had forgotten. At ground level

there is no resemblance. Next time you chat
with your next-door neighbour, you are relieved
to find that you don't fancy him.

A week later you meet your ex-lover
at a party, after more than a year.
He reminds you (although only slightly)
of your next-door neighbour. He has a paunch
like your neighbour's before he went on that diet.
You remember how much you despise him.

He behaves as if he's pleased to see you.
When you leave (a little earlier
than you'd intended, to get away)
he gives you a kiss which is more than neighbourly
and says he'll ring you. He seems to mean it.
How odd! But you are quite relieved
to find that you don't fancy him.

Unless you do? Or why that sudden
something, once you get outside
in the air? Why are your legs prancing
so cheerfully along the pavement?
And what exactly have you just remembered?
You go home cursing chemistry.

Eileen Duggan

The Boastful Lover

If you should go in danger of a star,
    I would command its insolence to stand,
I'd make a ship to climb the silent sky,
    And pluck its burning core out with my hand.

If lightnings darted round your naked head—
    And oh, your head is haughty in these lands—
I'd turn your blinded eyes in to my breast,
    And catch the flying bolts with quiet hands.

Or if my foolish tongue your peril be,
    Though dear and close and secret are its bands,
I would go dumb and bleeding for your sake,
    And tear it from its roots with joyful hands.

But if the sight of me should be your dread,
  Be pitiful and try to understand.
I'll follow still and humble as a dog,
  Ah, do not spurn me with your little hand.

Brian Turner

Taking It as It Comes

I shrug off my shirt.
Burly men do it better, I'm sure,
but shrugging is manly

so I shrug away and cough,
pretending to clear my throat
just to be certain you notice me.

But I'm not nervous, no way.
He-men never are, not
in the presence of a mere woman.

I breathe deeply, in and out,
like a lifter preparing for his last attempt
at the snatch or a clean and jerk.

Now it's time for the shoes
that wink in the soft light
and look like trowels

peeping out from under the cuffs
of my nowhere near swanky trousers.
I slip off the shoes

and leave them well away from the bed
because, alas, they steam.
Next my strides. They drop

like a starting flag
and I have to concentrate hard
so as not to stumble and trip.

How I wish my legs were muscular,
lithe and brown with golden hairs
that whirred and twirled and tickled

and promised to twitch and firmly grip.
Again, alas, you've guessed,
they're not like that at all.

I slip my trousers over my feet
one leg at a time, and flip them aside.
Next the socks: I toe them aside, too,

and I'm nearly there. 'That's enough,'
you say, 'I want to do the rest.'
Ah, love of my life, sweet

athletic raunchy exotic
woman of my wildest wettest dreams,
where have you been hiding

all my agonising life?
Your skin is pale in the unimpeachable
moonlight and your teeth

gleam wickedly whenever you smile.
I give in, I say, if you promise
to eat me and keep me alive.

Hone Tuwhare

Mad

W. M.

I'm too early.
I wait the long slow minutes out,
my breath inheld, ready
to balloon up into a high, but for the slow
exhalation of my excitement as you turn
into the magic avenue of trees—your hand
held out to me—your hand

to my multiple infarctions—
awarenesses
of coin-silver leaves turning a-squint in air,
muffled footfalls on the footpath;
your naked ankles twinkling in the autumn light.
I close the distance between us
as quickly

as fog does boiling in
from the inner harbour inexorably
as the thunder and beat of train wheels
flashing past a tiny country station just
standing there   aghast   and quite
inexplicably shaken and lost and
without say.

Well, that is how you infect me: mad ay?

Denis Glover

Afterthought

Everything's right
Love or grief.
Your puzzled educated mind
In some ways ignorant of life
Makes me lovingly laugh.

Not cruelly, but enough.

Finality
I put in chosen banality
Words trivial but true—

I love you.

Peggy Dunstan

Looking Back

Twice
round the rotunda now
but still no place
to park
and even in the dark
it is not hard
to tell
the grass is littered
with love's aftermath
of latex.

Pale faces
swell and swim like fishes
in the under-water gloom.
Well,
does it matter?
We can go back
to our room—
It was stupid
of us anyway
to think we could recapture
that sated after-glance
of former rapture.

Albert Wendt

My Mother Dances

Through the shadows cast by the moon tonight
the memory of my mother dances
like the flame-red carp I watched
in the black waters of the lake
of the Golden Pavilion in Kyoto.
Such burning grace.

Though I am ill with my future
and want to confess it to her
I won't. Not tonight.
For my mother dances
in the Golden Pavilion
of my heart.

How she can dance.
Even the moon is spellbound
with her grace.

Jan Hutchison

My Mother and Father

And in old age too
she was excited by my

father. I could see it
in the kitchen.

The way her spoon slid
round the white sauce

then jigged as he spoke
her name. One time

she was sprinkling tips of
parsley in the steaming

broth, but stopped as
he walked through the door.

Her hands fluttered forward
in the air.

As if she held a ladle out
and it was spilling.

Russell Haley

Tannery Hill

I am beside myself
you sit alongside me
thinner than cobweb
a shape that only mind can hold
anonymous
but known
& there
& female—
you are the twelfth letter
of an unknown alphabet
a step I sometimes take
in darkness:

this is the valley
in which I used to ride—
these roads are new
the windmills were not there
before:
you have not spoken,
never speak,
but are
a form in the enclosed air;
I cannot hold the car
around this bend—
we leap into the trees.

Here I now hold you in
the perpetual moment of dying
    stay with me.

Fleur Adcock

Folie à Deux

They call it pica,
this ranging after alien tastes:
acorns (a good fresh country food,
better than I'd remembered)
that morning in the wood,

and moonlit roses—
perfumed lettuce, rather unpleasant:
we rinsed them from our teeth with wine.
It seems a shared perversion,
not just a kink of mine—

you were the one
who nibbled the chrysanthemums.
All right: we are avoiding something.
Tonight you are here early.
We seem to lack nothing.

We are alone,
quiet, unhurried. The whisky has
a smoky tang, like dark chocolate.
You speak of ceremony, of
something to celebrate.

I hear the church bells
and suddenly fear blasphemy,
even name it. The word's unusual
between us. But you don't laugh.
We postpone our ritual

and act another:
sit face to face across a table,
talk about places we have known
and friends who are still alive
and poems (not our own).

It works. We are altered
from that fey couple who talked out
fountains of images, a spray
of loves, deaths, dramas, jokes:
their histories; who lay

manic with words,
fingers twined in each other's hair
(no closer) wasting nights and hours;
who chewed, as dry placebos,
those bitter seeds and flowers.

It is the moment.
We rise, and touch at last. And now
without pretence or argument,
fasting, and in our right minds,
to go our sacrament.

Dinah Hawken

A Friend

She is lying beside another woman, a friend. They are talking together,
telling each other their dreams.
                              What a pleasure
holding hands, separate and together on the wide bed.
                              Now pleasure is turning
into joy, into kneeling together with their four hands
clasped like a strong heart. We have the whole world
in our hands, smiles one. What the hell
are we going to do with it, laughs the other.

Fiona Kidman

Pact for Mother and Teenager

Girl, we've quarrelled
in a motel in a strange town.
It's 2 a.m. and tomorrow
I'm due to drive north all day
on the holiday we've planned
this six months past.
If you were a lover,
I'd have thrown you out;
if you were your father,
I might have had a bitter-sweet
reconciliation. But as you are
my child, I watch you sleep
tangled in bedsheets and tearstains,
and try to plan the shortest way
out of town.

Jan Hutchison

Laura Sings to Her Corn-Cob Doll

Keep close to me
My corn-cob doll.
You have no eyes
You have no arms
And I must nurse
You carefully.

fa la la dee, my chickapea

Rock in my lap
Snug in your shawl
And you shall dream
Of sun and rain
And listen for
Cicadas' clap.

fa la la dee, my chickanap

I like your skin
With yellow doors.
Every one
Leads to a room.
It is your heart
Which sings 'Come in.'

fa la la dee, my chickapin

A Lesson on the Beach

A hood of shadows
gathers on this hill
but down on the beach

I can see you
properly. I measure
distances inside jagged

seams of sea and blue
heron sky. Love
is a loose shirt

which gives me room
to track the skid
of gulls' cries

and notice small
arrivals like these
pied stilts, crisp

in pink stockings
who yap and party
on the shore.

Now I trace your
sharp prints on the
sand's grey jacket

follow wind tunnels
through bent marram
grass. My lesson

isn't difficult.
I'm not needing
you today but dis

covering your
shine against rolled
leaves of taupata.

Ian Wedde

The Arrangement

With light across
your body: like

the peach
in a Cézanne dish

the glow seeming
to come from within,

softly, the skin
translucent,

fine down on it,
a crease for

the tongue
from

navel to
groin. Did

you arrange yourself
for such

effects, as Cézanne
his fruit upon the dish

his
painstaking *Nature*

Morte, or
was it

life, that quiet
accident.

Rachel McAlpine

Zig-Zag up a Thistle

1

A lot has changed here since the day
he left.
Fig trees have thrust up
their chubby fists,
tiny thumbs are dangling
from the sycamores,
cabbage tree's rococo
in her blonde embroidered plaits,
fuchsia bleeding pointedly
from every joint.

Some things remain the same:
the cat is happy.

And my fridge is over-full
of half-forgotten love,
marbled with islands of mould.

2

It's hard to fix your pronouns.
I was happy with 'me'.
Then we made an effort to be 'us'.
He retreated. I had to learn
'you' and 'him'.

I still say 'There are fig trees
in our street.'
I belong to many an us:
the family long and wide,
the human race.
Nobody lives alone.

Romans began their verbs incognito.
I (a part of us) got
two Christmas presents.
A Latin grammar once belonging
to my mother's grandmother.

A four-leafed clover
which I keep between
'idem, alius, alter, ceteri'
and 'hic, iste, ille, is'.

3

I used to have a friend and people said
how strong she was. I sanded
the banisters yesterday.
If only she were here! Her eyes
are nimble and her fingers slick
with putty, brush, plaster.

Today you touched my breast and so
I must be near. Thank you, thank you.
If I could find my friend
I might supervise your loving.

A final decision every day.
I check the calendar—
so far, thirty-two: nil.
Poetry's algebra,
love is arithmetic.
Some people say we are living
lives with a shape.

4

Sometimes you forget your lines
and have to act them out
again. This time,
should I flatter him, or cringe?

I have had such an urge to tidy up.
But I can work in a mess
and I usually do.

There is no
single perfect gesture,
and there is no amen.
The world will ad lib without end.

5

On a dry hill I look
at small brave lives.

A lark aspires to the orgasm
of a Pegasus. A ladybird
uses cocksfoot
for tightrope and trapeze.
Spiders zig-zag up a thistle.
Butterflies rely entirely
on their buoyant colours.

No one but the skylark travels
in a straight line.
The rest of us polka and pussyfoot.

6

The dandelion opens twice,
first to a dominant gold.
Then discarding petals
it clamps up tight,
and leggy seeds develop
in its grip.
And later—froth.

Love must change or die.
The future needs no feeding,
no permission.
It is white.
It happens somewhere else.

Love, work, children.
Angels fly on
two wings.

7

A good decision, that,
deciding to live, and properly.
Down on the beach it's hard to play
the tragedy queen for long.
Fathers watch their toddlers waddle,
lollipops laze in candy togs,
the sea explodes with kids
and yellow canoes.

You popping seed-pod of a world,
I love you, I love you,
let me come in!

Ian Wedde

2 for Rose

9

'If thy wife is small bend down to her & whisper in her ear' (Talmud)

                                        —what shall I
whisper?   that I dream it's no use any
more trying to hide my follies. If trees &

suchlike don't tell on me I understand
my son will & soon, too. His new blue eyes
see everything. Soon he'll learn to see
less. O the whole great foundation is sand.

But the drought has broken today, this rain!
pecks neat holes in the world's salty fabu-
lous diamond-backed carapace & doubt comes
out, a swampy stink of old terrapin.

What shall I say? 'I hid nothing from you,
but from myself. That I dream, little one,

10

by day & also by night & you are
always in the dream . . .' Oh you can get no
peace, will get none from me. The flower smells so
sweet who needs the beans? We should move house there
into the middle of the bean-patch: a
green & fragrant mansion, why not! Let's do
it all this summer & eat next year. O

let's tear off a piece. It's too hard & far
to any other dreamt-of paradise
& paradise is earthly anyway,
earthly & difficult & full of doubt.

I'm not good I'm not peaceful I'm not wise
but I love you. What more is there to say.
My fumbling voices clap their hands & shout.

Anton Vogt

For a Child's Drawing

This death-mask is my portrait by my son,
Whose childish eyes can trace the years' deep lines
Naively innocent of all they mean,
Shaping in shade what I had thought concealed.

Deftly his fingers find the flagging chin,
And fondly press the parted lips quite shut,
As if he feared that foolish words might spring
Prehensile from the hunger of my heart.

Lauris Edmond

Learning to Ride

Remember the sunlight tumbling
among the willows, the creaking of
saddles, the dust?—and round
the paddock, jolting and bouncing
the child, a brown knot tied, too
loose, on the nag's enormous shoulders
—the hands' fierce holding, the whole
small stubborn body shouting
determination not to fall . . .

It's a speaking body still, each
impulse defined in arch of bone or
pliant web of skin; see her twenty
years later wrenched by grief, head
bent to listen, arms to comfort
a helpless company; the hands that
mimed a child's resolve learn now
the solemn language of compassion.
Love in her is a steadiness of line,
a concentration in the eyes,
an angle, a spring held in the
flesh's taut dialectic.

Dear girl, when you ride again
let it be over round hills,
the cliffs not too close, let
your hands lie easily now
and under green willows
catkins fall on your hair.

C.K. Stead

Tall Girl

The tall girl with brown arms is walking
Between the elms in bluest evening,
Her breasts full of a melancholy sway,
Her face browner with the sun half-gone.

The tall girl is walking towards the hills.

She crosses a thin creek and rushy grass.
She crosses the line of my eyes that follow her,
And fades among the great breasts of the hills.

Hone Tuwhare

Annie

I am filled with your
richness and my remorse
(just now thickening
to a boil on my right ear)

I get down on my elbows
and knees, left . . . right,
left . . . right, painfully
picking up yesterday's apples
with my teeth; impossible.

But for my snot-shuffles
there is only a vast silence.
A space palpable and empty.

You've gone.
I read your note once more.
It is crumpled and smoothed
out again. You've gone. The
space you've left is
unbearable: I keep tripping
over it. Forgive me

but I do not want to lead
nor have you walk in front
and in my long shadow.

Come back. Walk on my
left side, heart-side; close:
the sun a noon-crown without
shadow

Rachel McAlpine

Before the Fall

After the bath with ragged towels
my Dad
would dry us very carefully:
six little wriggly girls,
each with foamy pigtails,
two rainy legs,
the invisible back we couldn't reach,
a small wet heart,
and toes, ten each.

He dried us all
the way he gave the parish
Morning Prayer:
as if it was important,
as if God was fair,
as if it was really simple
if you would just be still
and bare.

Alistair Te Ariki Campbell

August

Meeting my childhood love one day in magnificent
August, at the time when trees are wooed into leaf,
And conjuring ponds surprise the world with lilies
And wise-cracking ducks, when the green graminivorous
      Sun releases the snow-fettered hills

Into a myriad field-wandering, trespassing streams—
Her face, the shape of my heart; her mouth,
The guileless texture of the blackbird's song—
I hardly knew her for the frock she wore
      Of the colour of August, and her body

Loose as the wind-delighting poplar tree; stepping
So gaily out like a word from the cool white
Language of girls, my name so warm on her lips
And the day so rare, that from the cave-cool
       Band rotunda sweet sexual music

Straddled the wind-ruffled lake, and excited
The inhibited swan and drove him crazy,
And O, through foam of elder and cherry trees
The sparrows tumbled bewitched with song, with song—
       That love did not come to anything.

J.C. Beaglehole

You were Standing

You were standing by the honeysuckle
with the child in your arms,
and all that sunlit sweetness and your beauty
were linked entangled charms
to make a sudden long-remembered instant
in the sense-captured brain:
for you were fair like honeysuckle's flower
clothed in leaf-green again,
and the child in your arms was like a flower
opened after fresh rain.
You were smiling at the child with tenderness—
with a backward glance at me
you smiled too, and at your own carefulness
in new felicity.
It was like something I had seen already
but when I did not know—
long ago perhaps, or a dreamt vision
in sunlight long ago.
You went inside: I smelt the heavy sweetness
of bloom yellow and white
starred on the clustering climbing branches,
and it fixed in my sight
that moment recognised or dim-remembered
clearly seen at the last,
as you smiled at your awakened burden

like a part of the past
and future at once and the sun-drenched present;
with that backward glance too
smiling merrily at me you vanished.
And now always when you
are not in my sight I see you standing
smiling, holding the child
with a young conscious happy tenderness
and my mind is beguiled
as never before; but why does this picture
so blot every other?—
was it the sunlight on the honeysuckle
or thinking you a mother?

Lauris Edmond

Spring Afternoon, Dunedin

We lay in the long grass on the hill
high up near the crooked quince tree
and out of sight of the house.
The afternoon touched us with its
fragile sun—and then the mountain
suddenly reached up and took it.
So *early*—it was barely three
o'clock. Together we looked up

from our books and shivered,
then pulled up the rug and
hand in hand, talking of altitudes
and moons, we wandered home. Just so,
in a grass-sweet patch on a little
planet were we spinning minute by
minute out of our brightness and
into the changed, unloving years.

Hone Tuwhare

In October, Mary Quite Contemporary will be Seven Months Gone

Today she walks with the sun
friendly by her side
faking a coarse delight in
throwing a bulbous shadow on
a concrete wall

Obsequiously, the wind retreats
before the shifting surface
of polka dots and bumps that is
her spinnaker-dress

Sun-wreathed, her face quirks
a Mona Lisa: for tomorrow
her plump majesty shall wear
a crown of pain to His coming

Eileen Duggan

The Bushfeller

Lord, mind your trees to-day!
My man is out there clearing.
God send the chips fly safe.
My heart is always fearing.

And let the axehead hold!
My dreams are all of felling.
He earns our bread far back.
And then there is no telling.

If he came home at nights,
We'd know, but it is only—
We might not even hear—
A man could lie there lonely.

God, let the trunks fall clear,
He did not choose his calling;
He's young and full of life—
A tree is heavy, falling.

Nick Williamson

Making Love

We are past making children
but if we join together
we can make the stars
fall from the sky.

Sam Hunt

Cuckold Song

We are not allowed to
Your old man's told you—
Don't ever trust that guy,
The one with freckled knees
A stutter and a sly
Old dog called Blue Vein Cheese.

But here we are together
Caught in carnal weather
Without a coat without
In fact a bloody stitch
Ready for another bout
Your marriage in the ditch.

Your husband was a cuckold
First time I saw your face
Days before we ever rolled
That man took second place.

Those prayers you know by heart—
Get down on bended knee
Pray he finds it in his heart
Forgive you girl for loving me.

Get back to your marriage
Back to your tidy man,
Forget your grief, your rage,
Who you are, who I am.

Meg Campbell

The Way Back

Often we strayed far into the woods,
like those children in the folk tale,
but we always found our way back.
You were older, and I
simply followed behind you,
leaving you to think for both of us
(I was conditioned to follow
an older child). But listen—
it was I who thought to drop pebbles,
I, alone, who recognised the witch
in all her guises. I who pushed her
into her oven and pulled you from the cage,
and together we picked our way home
from pebble to pebble, while you said
it was me you really loved,
and I believed you,
knowing that you were wise.

Russell Haley

The Dogs/The Face

for Susie

you are lonely
lonely
your husband is tripping
says you are ugly:

outside in the yard
I opened the barn doors
one pair to each wall
I have lodged them at right-angles:

we lie down as easily as children
listen to the black dogs

howling in the barn—
they tug against their ropes
strain out
through
the doors:

I am
this house
this family
dismantling a beam
I smile at men in cassocks—
the dwarf who nurses a swollen hand
is mine: he covers his lap
with green leaves:

we own nothing
rent this space
these open walls—

Anne French

Three Love Poems

1

If you were dead, or had gone away for ever
to a distant place I could not visit, I
think I could contrive a modus vivendi.
Nothing glorious or vivid, just a competent,

honourable, decent manner of living. But
you are here; alive, yes, and tolerably
happy; I could dial a number this minute
and hear your voice answer. The distance

between us has shrunk from a metaphorical
few thousand miles to an actual six or seven.
Yet for all my tears, and despair, for all
time's passing, it seems I have progressed

no further than this manifest incapacity
not to love you, or forget, not to want
to hold you in my arms, and touch your face
with my fingers, and say your name.

2

The unspeakable truth
is that you, who could,
do not choose

me; and I who would
choose you
cannot choose not to.

3

In the end, whatever 'end' may mean,
you will turn into an old man; and
in the long run we will both be dead.

My love for you will not be recalled
in any obituary. The panegyric delivered
over your corpse will make no mention

of my name; no mason will engrave
it with yours in granite, entwined
in hearts—'They are in death united

(as they were not in life)'. Nor will
your widow spill the beans (what beans?)
to your biographer. Letters will be lost

or burned, poems will be wilfully misread;
dates will be forgotten, messages we wrote
each other on the flyleaf of a dozen books

will be misconstrued; and our friends,
who can be relied upon to do their best,
will get the facts completely wrong.

Supposing there's no one who'll recall
my love for you when we are dead: then
let these words stand as its memorial.

Charles Brasch

To C.H. Roberts

I set your name upon the page, but have no words
To express what silence best perhaps can say,
Unless I borrow Dante's to the shades
Of mount and ditch—*così com'io t'amai* . . .
m'insegnavate come . . . and by such oblique
But unequivocal testimony declare
What I recall, wondering as I look back,
Our lives' dear dialogue now in its twentieth year:
A dialogue distance cannot end nor time,
Yawn as they will between our worlds, for you
Are never silent in me, never seem
Less near than when I watched you and longed to grow
Your equal; because no day, no night can come
That does not bring some echo of a word or thought
Once ours; because we are that mortal ground
The spiritual and temporal powers dispute,
And I still turn towards you when I cannot stand
Alone, as in those years that are most my theme,
Oxford, Soulbury, Llanthony, Trier, Venice, Kôm Aushim.

Ruth Gilbert

Even in the Dark

As a room you know
And, entering at midnight,
Walk through effortlessly—
By sense not sight
Passing unscathed between
Table and chair,
Eluding the low footstool,
Faultlessly aware
Of bowl and ledge,
Of flower and fluted vase,

Coming unerringly
Without fear or pause
To the desk with its waiting book,
Paper-knife, and bookmark:

As this room I would have you know me
Even in the dark.

Adrienne Jansen

A Poem of Farewell

What is left to say?
All the large words
have been spoken.

I'd take one of the
smallest words, like love,
wrap it in a warm breath,
tie it with a knot of flax,
and leave it, nonchalantly,
on your papers.

A small green leaf
among the river stones.

Don't throw it out
by accident, or crush it.
Slip it in your pocket,
where its touch
might sometimes
warm your fingers.

Connections

You are part of my mind,
that deep quiet sea
which sleeps, blue on blue,
under the rattle and jarring
of hours and faces colliding.

You float, and in moments
of slow welling silence, I join you.

We drift, without touching.

Sam Hunt

Those Eyes; Such Mist

Sea mists from the upper inlet
lift, the morning hills afloat.

I dream of the several men who've
sailed seven seas; their many mists;

wake again to your love
as thick dreams clear; a dream of masts,

a dream that no man ever
saw your eyes like this.

I have lost all voice. I kiss
those eyes, our voyaging; such mist.

Robin Healey

Pullover

I want to be your little black sleeveless pullover
so I can feel your ribs
pout gently for your boobs
sit neatly at your waist
and as you see yourself in glass as you pass

I can ask in a neatly knitted way
how you like me now dear sweet coz.

And then at night when, ah, you ease me
over your head, flicking your clean
shiny hair as I go, you can fling me
into your chair. I'll lie about
all vee neck, armholes and contentment
hoping for a cold morning
and a warm wool ride all day long.
Smell me, I smell of you, think of me as stylish,
wear me into holes, cherish me, cherish me.

M.K. Joseph

Romeo and Juliet (Duet)

The river runs the mountains sing
Into the hollow dome of night
The stars into the fountain fling
A palm and pinnacle of light
Tender shall be our loving
In all the bodied dark and bright.
  Soft and shining is my love
  As the orient fruit in the orange grove.

While water's melancholy song
Drowns a midnight of alarms
And the moonmoth with enchanted tongue
About the honeysuckle swarms
This golden child all the night long
Hangs summer lightning in my arms.
  Quick and sheer is my darling
  As the swallow on the wing.

We are life's minions and the lords
(Clothed in a dark and scented air)
Of death's dominion, of the sword's
Whistling edge, the graying hair
The dull weight of ambiguous words
Successive generations bear.
  Incorporate, we two in one
  Beatify the summer dawn.

The hairy shepherds drowse in dream
Of clouds that pasture on the hill
The haycocks glisten by the stream
And chanticlere and skylark shrill.
Arm and breast and forehead gleam
Like marble to the morning's chill
   Bedded in the pallid gloom
   Two effigies upon a tomb.

Betty Bremner

Versions

She knew so much about love—
Heloise and Abelard—
was there ever
such a passion as theirs,
Tristan and Iseult
asleep in the forest
with the sword between,
Antony who gazed wide-eyed
on the great Egyptian Queen
and cried
the half has not been told me!
Don Quixote who loved
pure and chaste from afar
his Dulcinea,
Porgy and Bess,
and many lesser lovers
timeless between the covers.

But when he came
she discovered that love
was like facing into the sun
the dazzle
almost took her breath away
and was, she said,
quite unlike
the love in books.

Rachel Bush

You Wouldn't Read About It

It hasn't all been roses.
You've got to take the rough with
the smooth. 'Marry me,' he said.
So I did. We still have a
good laugh over that. Well as
long as you've still got your sense of
humour as the bishop
said to the chorus girl Ha ha.
Do you know it? The one about the oh no
I really shouldn't. You'll think
I'm awful. And some of it's
been too good to be true. No
offence meant but you wouldn't
believe some of the things we
get up to like
        one substantial mortgage
        producing three lovely kids
        growing some of our own vegies
        filling out IR12s
        Rotary dos
        camping at Pohara after Boxing Day
        buying Chinese on Fridays
        (it used to be fish and chips)
        watching our arches drop
        losing our hair or dyeing it.
Only what I keep
thinking is I mean
I just wonder you know
could this be the experience
of a lifetime?

Gary McCormick

Time

In the time I have known you, you have grown taller, thinner,
like a willowy tree whose roots have drunk too long
from the waters of a cool, clear stream.
Whose knowledge comes from higher places.
The mountains perhaps,
where the air is sharp and clear and flowers grow
hugging the stone.
That feeling of distance, of looking up at you, may have been
part of the attraction, part of the mystery.

When I am coming back, all I can think about
is you; the drinking, the thinking and the good life.
How you move on your own and when we
are together, we have no need
of talk. A glance can take an hour and a smile between us
travels like light.
I have fought against it; I don't know anybody who has walked
more miles, been left standing, cried, shouted, grown angry, been
left wondering: why this, why you, why me?

You have spoken of cowboys, things left suspended,
of travel through time, temporary blindness.
We are the lucky ones; not because of what we have
but for the knowledge of what we lack.
I have you to thank for it, your delicate beauty
shining through against the light.
You have shown me what can be taken away, all movement
is small, the veins of a petal once bursting with love,
outlines its passing.

I have decided to go on falling,
to make my way, not by design, but by following
the careless light love gives by way of gravity.

Cilla McQueen

A Lightning Tree

my wild love seeks a fastening place
but passion kills with heaviness
I want to give you tenderness
not deadly electricity

so I have made of words a lightning tree
to earth my dangerous love through poetry.

Wild Sweets

what I mean by
love? a terrorist incident
a torn artery an electric arc a
touch without fear
hand in a flame
leather seduction cup of tea
curly rose cushion scrambled eggs
stroke wheel stomp stiletto
in the arch of the foot
spearing the bones
sucking wild sweets
without word talk, it's
not that I love for any at all
thing to get from you
but my learning to cease
expectation.

Heather McPherson

Be Quiet

Be quiet, heart.
And stop this shaking, hands.
She hasn't come to stay—

nothing you say is what she wants to know.
Keep still, I say!
And talk, if you must, of gardens.

Ask if she saw the poppies at the gate—
tell her the last cutting's doing fine—
you've watered it and finger it for buds.
You've dug through twitch and dragged
convolvulus from its writhed nest round
the iris to lie, white hairless worms
in the concrete sun.

Say it's a long job—soil so veined resists
a thorough sifting—one tendril and it crawls again
up fence, tree, window, walls—
say anything—
say you saw a seagull caught by a gust
tip backwards till its wings arched and it caught
the upward break—
say the garden's haunted—
one shadow in the corner doesn't change—
feet walk up the path and no-one's there—
but laugh it off.

Don't say you lie in the dark and stare
while the clock beats crazy paving in your head
and the pruned rose knocks a nailless finger
on the glass.
Down, tremor. Say nothing when she speaks—
nothing she couldn't put in a bag of coloured stones
to, one day, make a border.

Never—however blooming, budding, dead, say: Stay.
The bag might tear, the poppies wilt, the cutting
split in half—suckers might slide under the path
and choke out shooting bulbs. Or
she might go
saying no.

Her tone's too kind? Thin blinds drop in her eyes
and leave you seagull space?
Burn harder, heart.
Don't wince. Don't turn away.

Bill Manhire

The Kiss

The damp sky is eating your hair.
The day drags its branches over.
There is no beautiful rest in which
you can do no wrong. Give me the teeth,
says the universe. You are neither here
nor there, but walking.

The direction you are taking
cries a low welcome
and darkness sinks its bone
in your shoulder. Under the stars
you are fed somewhat on stars.
Their popular wounds light your body.

A tale of grasslands under the sky.
A tale of hesitation.
The tale of a woman, pressing
her breasts against the window.
A tale of hesitation.
A tale of grasslands under the sky.

City Life

Rainy days inside
We starved and fell in love
Small bird
Let's sit here on the roof
And make some decisions about the city

The sandpit's big enough to sleep in
Days and days
With nothing to talk about
Till we both slipped out of the house together
I still can't believe it

Wings and stalks, see how they fly
Our life together under some stairs
Some moonlight entering
Large flowers that last in a jar
Well where will we go from there?

Damp afternoons, the darkness in the garden
Remember I followed you home by night
So tired and turning over
And going at last to sleep then
Not loving you less, but better

Elizabeth Nannestad

The Kiss

There we were—two people
and a lot of scenery.

I don't know what business
you had to kiss me—now

everyone is interested:
the low boughs of pohutukawa

the shoulders of sand and the marram,
our radiant moon.

Don't stop now—think
how we'd disappoint them.

Against Housework

I don't know why our friends say there's no room
where we live. We keep bringing in more
books and flowers, there must be room.
One of these days, if the spiders go on spinning
and we do no work at all
we won't be able to see out, we'll be spun in.

One by one the animals outside
lean on the step where normally I clean my shoes.
Their noses leave a spot of wet.
It's not that we don't admit anyone

but we do forget, occupied with the uncharted land
across the sheets: mountains sliding away—
your knees. My untidy love, my sloven. Here we drank eternity
and for us, it was ordinary.

Alistair Paterson

from *What Never Happened*

5

Waking in the dark and knowing you sleep
somewhere far off, I light a cigarette,
listen for the beating of your heart,
the sounds of your breathing,
and remember I cannot turn to you again
for the violence of love,
those paroxysms of that secret art
your body made beautiful on that last day
when the sun saw us part.

                        I see you in water,
where mountains grope in cloud for rain,
hear your voice above the fluting of the wind,
recollect nights that made you beautiful,
how your long and loving limbs, smooth arms
unbent and seemed mysteriously to grow
more passionate than dawn on gleaming snow,
remember the way your body moved
in accordance with a language of its own,
its secret syntax and vocabulary—
gerunds, nouns, adjectives and verbs.

Here in the dark, I remember the shape
of what you are and the ways; no longer
knowing how to say what eyes could
and hands, I count the nights
we once owned, the mornings and the days.

Iain Sharp

Owed to Joy

Three years after we were first an item
Joy wants to know why
I've never used her name in poems.

Really it's just an old student's fear
of being thought portentous—
like Lucifer in *Paradise Lost*

farewelling happy fields (where Joy
forever dwells!)—or Doc Johnson
fixing his great jowls against Vanity

and other upper-case Temptations.
Styles change. Though keen still to seem sage-like,
the writers we actually know

offer their advice with lowered voices.
Passion, according to Albert, lasts
only six months. Now, warns Sheridan,

when what was once an electric secret
becomes the norm, the hard work begins.
Yes, it's difficult, but I still feel passionate

and walking together today in Cornwall Park
down Twin Oaks Drive—the lambs lying languorous
after their first shearing, the pohutukawas

redder than I've ever dreamed (though perhaps
I say that every year) and the sky
an unstoppable blue prairie—I want

to call out 'Joy! Joy! Joy!' and not give a damn
who mistakes me for someone happy
to the point of abstraction.

Vivienne Plumb

I Love Those Photos

I love those photos I took in '79 in the desert,
all sky, red sand and dust at sunset.
And one gum leaf pressed flat in a book,
curled like a crescent moon
pink and green. Last night, I dreamt
I broke it, the smell of eucalyptus
crumbling in my hand.
Me making homemade jam, marmalade
and relish, glowing like fists of jelly
jewels in clean clear jars.
And that night we stayed up really late,
got drunk, and thought we might
ring up people we hate and
make funny noises down the phone.
I laughed, and then we lit the candles again
on your birthday cake, and you bent forward
and blew, and then it was black,
and in the darkness, I just touched you.

Gregory O'Brien

Tall Woman Story II

Marlborough Sounds, May 1994

A day will only hold
so much

      then it will start
dropping things. Like the waves

it will accommodate us,
      the deckchair out on
its verandah of wind, the travelling world

      lapping
at the edge of the Sounds. These mysteries
of light,
      and the dark

we know everything
about. In the quiet, smaller
                hours, the wedding ring

announces itself on
the sides of pools or vessels.
                Enclosed by it, warmed

even, we have made the ring
a home. The bay has drawn up
                a contract. Between

table and tree, the ring
rolls down a cold path.
                You catch it

on your finger, the second finger
from the left, the one
                that steers the boat

most, that most
grips the warm
                tiller.

Roma Potiki

Incognito

I was just looking and smiling
I didn't mean anything by it
of course—

but who was I to say no
when you walked over
and parked yourself and yr bags
next to my leg?

The Franz Joseph Glacier was awesome.
I love New Zealand. I'm coming back y'know.

That's just what all the tourist boys
say isn't it?

I laughed
you looked a bit nervous
I thought—
and so skinny
like the wind would blow you
out into the harbour and float
you driftwood-like
into the wide embrace of
Te Moana Nui a Kiwa.

Haa! We breathed the same breath
and it was night,
a long night
and then slowly day
and the breath mingled
and bodies became one mass.
We bayed and rolled
an international language.

I could see the old ladies screeching and cawing
like rock'n'roll
and over-the-thigh hip-hop
and cheeky with it too.

Why not if you're able?

We certainly were a pair
of tumbling accoutrements
exchanging
life experience and
the most exquisite music
for nothing at all
but each other
and the wonderful adagio
of rustling movement
and exemplary, tousled
dishevelment.

I know
we shan't be making beds together.

I'm sure it's someone else's job.

I searched for a long espresso
on a cold, pelting start to a day.

You wanted tea, a gentler drug,

Addicted to the place.

Alan Riach

A Poem about Four Feet

Last night, my two feet
lay on each other, warm as toast
in my single bed, between clean sheets,
till I rose, padded over
the New Zealand wool carpet to
the kitchen linoleum, sat down
at the table, and wrote
about your two feet in your socks,
tramping somewhere north of the equator,
in the middle of my night.
I was thinking of how my two feet
had lain there sleeping,
folded, like cats, twitching,
wondering, where your two feet,
which wanted them to play with,
were. And how they would have been
so much happier
sleeping near to each other,
four familiar feet,
hard, soft and warm,
in a single bed
somewhere, with you, alone.

Bill Sewell

Aubade

Awake before dawn; and it's not natural to
rise in the dark. The birds aren't to blame,
up and about and disgustingly keen, nor
the curtains with their transparency. No,
it's the weight; and you'd think it would
lift with the light. And don't say, *ah,
there's somebody with him!* Would that

it were as easy as saying goodbye,
throwing a last look at her snowy skin.
But no one and nothing is leaving now,
though the birds may twitch and complain.
There's no crusade or possessive father
to drag me away. It's this weight deadening
inside, waking me up to remind me.

Keith Sinclair

Girl Loved by the Moon

Watching your face asleep is very strange
like daylight visits to the landscape of my dreams;
as if among a crowd my fantasies
were acted out in some prolonged charade;
so strange, your face, so utterly,
and in this deep repose like someone else's,
someone I've never known, perhaps a boy's,
or someone known too well, not quite forgotten—
wax image of my mother as a girl.
You belong to the moon now and milky ways
where I cannot walk awake.
Opening my eyes I think such things
and ask myself if I have loved before
since loving you is like a dictionary
opened at random on words I never knew,
or never knew I knew.
Seeing your so beloved face recast
by night's most clever, gentle fingers
and sunk, deep, utterly, in a youthful calm
pushes new roads through tuff and scoria
of ordinary living by clock and rule,
to streams of melting snow, tall peaks of noon
on a long drive to wide dramatic country,
the glare, the sexual blare of summer
and shadowed afternoon, naked beneath trees.
Now the moon peers coldly through venetian blinds and tries to take you.
I dare, I dare stand up to my pale rival.
I hit, I hold, hold hard, I call you back,

back to our lips and limbs
intertwined like trade winds and the tropics.

So you awake and in your opening eyes
I see my life wrapped up in dreamy paper.

James K. Baxter

He Waiata Mo Te Kare

1

Up here at the wharepuni
That star at the kitchen window
Mentions your name to me.

Clear and bright like running water
It glitters above the rim of the range,
You in Wellington,
I at Jerusalem,

Woman, it is my wish
Our bodies should be buried in the same grave.

2

To others my love is a plaited kono
Full or empty,
With chunks of riwai,
Meat that stuck to the stones.

To you my love is a pendant
Of inanga greenstone,
Too hard to bite,
Cut from the boulder underground.

You can put it in a box
Or wear it over your heart.

One day it will grow warm,
One day it will tremble like a bed of rushes
And say to you with a man's tongue,
'Taku ngakau ki a koe!'

3

I have seen at evening
Two ducks fly down
To a pond together.

The whirring of their wings
Reminded me of you.

4

At the end of our lives
Te Atua will take pity
On the two whom he divided.

To the tribe he will give
Much talking, te pia and a loaded hangi.

To you and me he will give
A whare by the seashore
Where you can look for crabs and kina
And I can watch the waves
And from time to time see your face
With no sadness,
Te Kare o Nga Wai.

5

No rafter paintings,
No grass-stalk panels,
No Maori mass,

Christ and his Mother
Are lively Italians
Leaning forward to bless,

No taniko band on her head,
No feather cloak on his shoulder,

No stairway to heaven,
No tears of the albatross.

Here at Jerusalem
After ninety years
Of bungled opportunities,
I prefer not to invite you
Into the pakeha church.

6

Waves wash on the beaches.
They leave a mark for only a minute.
Each grey hair in my beard
Is there because of a sin,

The mirror shows me
An old tuatara,
He porangi, he tutua,
Standing in his dusty coat.

I do not think you wanted
Some other man.

I have walked barefoot from the tail of the fish to the nose
To say these words.

7

Hilltop behind hilltop,
A mile of green pungas
In the grey afternoon
Bow their heads to the slanting spears of rain.

In the middle room of the wharepuni
Kat is playing the guitar,—
'Let it be! Let it be!'

Don brings home a goat draped round his shoulders.
Tonight we'll eat roasted liver.

One day, it is possible,
Hoani and Hilary might join me here,
Tired of the merry-go-round.

E hine, the door is open,
There's a space beside me.

8

Those we knew when we were young,
None of them have stayed together,
All their marriages battered down like trees
By the winds of a terrible century.

I was a gloomy drunk.
You were a troubled woman.
Nobody would have given tuppence for our chances,
Yet our love did not turn to hate.

If you could fly this way, my bird,
One day before we both die,
I think you might find a branch to rest on.

I chose to live in a different way.

Today I cut the grass from the paths
With a new sickle,
Working till my hands were blistered.

I never wanted another wife.

9

Now I see you conquer age
As the prow of a canoe beats down
The plumes of Tangaroa.

You, straight-backed, a girl,
Your dark hair on your shoulders,
Lifting up our grandchild,

How you put them to shame,
All the flouncing girls!

Your face wears the marks of age
As a warrior his moko,
Double the beauty,
A soul like the great albatross

Who only nests in mid-ocean
Under the eye of Te Ra.

You have broken the back of age.
I tremble to see it.

10

Taraiwa has sent us up a parcel of smoked eels
With skins like fine leather.
We steam them in the collander.
He tells us the heads are not for eating,

So I cut off two heads
And throw them out to Archibald,
The old tomcat. He growls as he eats
Simply because he's timid.

Earlier today I cut thistles
Under the trees in the graveyard,
And washed my hands afterwards,
Sprinkling the sickle with water.

That's the life I lead,
Simple as a stone,
And all that makes it less than good, Te Kare,
Is that you are not beside me.

Part 3

The heart has no corners

Alistair Paterson

Jennie Roache Love All the Boys in the World

Who are you Jennie and how do you look
are your eyes rounded blue does your hair
tumble or twine do you have cheeks
curved and full and when you smile
do your lips incline ruefully down
are you the child in every woman the
one who runs water through her hands
and watches as if water were new
her hands unknown who cannot touch
plum apple grape or peach
without experiencing fulsome pleasures
roundness smoothness roughness taste
do you sleep at night then wake
hugging the dark as if it were a friend
conscious of the liberties you take
and are your stars so bright they want
no polishing are you sad enough sometimes
to know that happiness always borrows
that nothing it owns is ever kept
have you dolls and do you read books
do you bake or cook take singing lessons
ever pause just to sit and look
listen to other children play who
taught you and how did you learn to spell
where could you have got so early soon
years before such facts are due your
fragment of the truth how could you have
laughed so much wept long enough to know
that there's flesh beyond your flesh
and bone beyond your growing bone where
did you learn of the need Jennie Roache
and what was the impulse prompted you
to write your declaration on my fence?

Elizabeth Nannestad

We Watched the Moon Rise

We watched the moon rise
above the line of mountains.
The night was ice and sharp stars
and we shivered, my head on your shoulder.
We waited until the moon
was fully come, large and yellow
then went to our beds
and the moon
took the short way
around and went back down.

Harry Ricketts

How Things Are

This is how things are:
if you leave their mother
the likelihood is you'll lose your kids.

Of course you love them;
they're the heart of your life.
This is how things are.

Should you stay till they're
older, then go? You know
the likelihood is you'll lose your kids.

You'd write, send presents.
They'd never understand.
This is how things are.

Each day it just gets
worse. Look, you're going under.
The likelihood is you'll lose your kids.

You may or may not
be to blame. It's the same.
This is how things are:
the likelihood is you'll lose your kids.

Harry Ricketts

Under the Radar

Wordsworth knew a thing or two
about suffering: how it's
'permanent, dark and obscure
And shares the nature of infinity.'

True enough; though he doesn't
mention how little one can
do for oneself—let alone
for others. Always under your radar

and you under mine, we know
the darker frequencies by heart.
Sometimes we seem two ghosts
obscurely haunting each other's lives.

James Norcliffe

Easy Thai Cooking

the canned rambutans
are stuffed with pineapple

the syrup is as thin and sweet
as the waitresses with their
thin legs and sweet smiles
who hover nervously while
waiting for the puzzling orders

the television on the wall is loud
with primary colours and kickboxing

our waitress is very pregnant
I wonder about the effect of hot
chilli prawns on the unborn child

and I remember the way you would
take my hand and place it on the white
bowl of your belly to feel the fish-nibble
butting of our babies' fists and feet

there is a necessary breeze from the fan
which lifts your hair slightly and fills
the room with lemongrass and garlic

and all at once the world is a place
of billowing and butting as sharp
and sweet briefly as the crisp chilli
catfish with the tamarind sauce

expert with chopsticks I watch as you
carefully pick out all of your slippery
button mushrooms to put on my plate

it makes me smile and reach out
and the waitress hurries over
to ask if I need anything else

In the Food Court

the power of love first falls
like a powdery condiment
all over the grilled tiger prawns
in black pepper sauce

its presence in the air
alerts somnambulant diners
and they pause in mid-fork
& look about with widening eyes
through love-filled shafts of sunlight

I see their pin-striped shirts
and button-down collars
slowly swell with the power of love

& while they wait the power of love
fills the whole room as if it were
a large bowl of fine blue china
& love sways there aromatic
spicy splashing this way and that

then with a dying burst of static
the music fades into shadows
and might never have been
were it not for the young woman
at the next table dabbing
a blood-red drip of *tom yam*
from the white shirt of her lover

Katherine Mansfield

He Wrote

Darling Heart if you would make me
Happy, you have found the way.
Write me letters. How they shake me
Thrill me all the common day

With our love. I hear your laughter
Little laughs! I see your look
'They Lived Happy Ever After'
As you close the faery book.

Work's been nothing but a pleasure
Every silly little word
Dancing to some elfin measure
Piped by a small chuckling bird.

All this love—as though I've tasted
Wine too rare for human food—
I have dreamed away and wasted
Just because the news was good.

Where's the pain of counting money
When my little queen is there
In the parlour eating honey
Beautiful beyond compare!

How I love you! You are better.
Does it matter—being apart?
Oh, the love that's in this letter
Feel it, beating like a heart.

Beating out—'I do adore you'
Now and to Eternity
See me as I stand before you
Happy as you'd have me be.

Lauris Edmond

Those Roses

Roses, the single scarlet sort,
open at the throat as if for
coolness, sprawl at the window;
you heap on my plate a pile
of potatoes, steaming and small,
smelling of mint. 'They're
basic,' you say as we go at them
lustfully, 'they grow by the door;
you have to chase meat'—and I
notice a certain vegetable poise,
not striated like the fibrous
deposits of a more strenuous growing
but smooth, opaque; placid testimony
to the sufficiency of flesh.

'Of course you do have to hunt—'
I say, thinking of hopeful
burrowings in the soil, wresting
from the clutch of its black fingernails
each creamy nugget; and we agree
on that; we're a bit languid,
munching more slowly as each
pale pod splits open and fills
us with amber warmth—one flesh
sturdily giving itself to another.
Those roses, too, they lean over us,
and the squat black pot gives
off its dull gleam, grinning
crookedly from the stove.

Harvey McQueen

To Anne

Our foolish cat patiently
watched me cut liver into
catsized pieces, then as
I dropped it to her dish

sprinted out the open back
door to sit mewing at the
closed front door waiting
for me to let her in. Cats
rightly enter with style.

Think sometimes I act like
that, not accepting what
you abundantly offer without
creating needless difficulty.

Harvey McQueen

At Ease

Today
like an old dog
sleeping all over
the furniture
I feel comfortable.

You rang

& your letter
arrived
you wrote on grey paper
but sounded cheerful.

Good
we should be cheerful.

Last night
my forked body
watched the detached moon
slowly come clean
from the clouds.

Most of the time
I act out
the images of others.

In your presence
I feel at ease
& generous
like my old friend the sun.

By flesh we share the same community.

George Sweet

The Shopping List

She writes down that
they are out of butter.
She writes it on the Shopping List.
All week there is no entry from him.

She invites his friends for dinner.
He dresses with care, muttering,
because the shirt he prefers is
in the wash.

He comments.
She coaches him about the
laundry basket.

He discovers, muttering,
that there is no wine.

She says that she got some
from the supermarket.
It's in the fridge, chilling.

She coaches him about the
Shopping List.

They seek counselling.
He know not why.
She weeps.
He knows not why.

She takes out the family cheque book,
and pays for the session.

R.A.K. Mason

Footnote to John ii 4

Don't throw your arms around me in that way:
　　I know that what you tell me is the truth—
　　yes I suppose I loved you in my youth
　　as boys do love their mothers, so they say,

but all that's gone from me this many a day:
I am a merciless cactus an uncouth
wild goat a jagged old spear the grim tooth
of a lone crag . . . Woman I cannot stay.

Each one of us must do his work of doom
and I shall do it even in despite
of her who brought me in pain from her womb,
whose blood made me, who used to bring the light
and sit on the bed up in my little room
and tell me stories and tuck me up at night.

James K. Baxter

Mill Girl

Attendant angel, mark this one
Fresh as paint in the flower of her sixteenth year:
With sheltering wing surround her. The great loom she
Tends, like a monstrous child—its bellowings stun,
Drug, drown her mind like the drumming of a weir;
Her heart's yet innocent of time's captivity.

Nor does she see behind the eyes that feed
On her rose, rash nubility (the tough boys
Who yarn, mending the broken bobbin-strings)
A tigerish jungle of incontinent need,
A cobra's nonchalance swaying at poise,
A bar room vanity that blinks and springs.

She waits in the ignorant garden of her wishes
Till Mr Right (first glimpsed in *The Oracle*) come
Darkhaired and smiling to take her ungloved hand
And lead her into a world lovely as fishes,
Secret as starlight, out of the stagnant slum
She knows, the flyspecked kitchen, to a table at the Grand.

Though Love cannot save, at least it will watch and weep
On that near night when she, under a moonless sky
On wet park leaves, or on a mattress in a back
Room at the party, loses what none can keep—
Rough and ready, before the keg runs dry
Fumbled and forced—yet willing, ready to learn the knack.

W.H. Oliver

Peacocks

Strangely in this suburb peacocks constantly cry
strutting behind their wire. If there were tended
lawns sloping to a docile river, if an antique
decorum was defined when the birds shrieked
and displayed flamboyant sexual colours to the eyes
of gentlepeople pacing gravelled paths
who in such ways were minded of the other
uses for the languorous summer half-light . . .
no mullioned windows mask unambiguous ardours
discreetly managed behind closed curtains.
Still, the birds shriek and exhibit the colours
of appetite and desire; within the weatherboard houses
there's passion enough. Though the decorum has departed
the curtains are strictly drawn and the nights are close.

Kendrick Smithyman

This Blonde Girl

This blonde girl carries sorrow on her shoulder
and all my world swings at her fingertips
darkness and light, while red as a berry her lips
make marks of music on me that never colder
the legendary spheres may equal. She will sing
through every ocean chapel of my being
and bird be of my eye at waking morning,
perched on the twig of a time will never stop.

And if I come to her it is to tell
how she inhabits me and moves like water
through these intrinsic habits and may rove
freelance of my whole image now and later,
having walked innocent in wonder and in all
of harm familiar, grown up again to love.

Iain Lonie

Mirror Language

We can't go on meeting like this
or in this place: the dark
acrid hotel corridor
with its mirror at the far end

never knowing whether this time
it's to be farce or melodrama: who
will I see in the mirror, Groucho
or the woman in white?

I say: it must end sometime, I
have a life to get on with, but you—
and as soon as I say it, lip-read
the mirror's answer in mirror language

complaining 'What would I do all day?
There's nowhere to go: it's so boring here
and besides
you couldn't get on without me.'

Oh mirror language is so banal
and everything it says is true:
with us, it can never be
tragedy or comedy: we pad

the length of the commonplace
like a carpet damp underfoot
and turn and pad back again
but do we want to be free?

Why, as soon as I suggest it, the
tinnitus of nightmare begins
the pursuit through silence and dark: 'How
can I live

if you hide yourself from me?'
to the meeting at some nowhere
with your pale-lipped reproach: 'Why
did you kill my love dead?'—fictions

which leave us with nothing to invent.
We need each other, as the themes
of tragedy need each other:
love facing death in the mirror

M.K. Joseph

For My Children

To you who have come
In this tired time
Ruled not by stars
But by two wars

What can we give
Excepting love
That having no end
Pays no dividend?

And what bequeath
But island earth
From Eden yet
Whole seas apart?

But still the spring
Renews its song
Immortal life
Through bud and leaf

And so we pray
No cliff too high
No gulf too deep
For hand and hope.

Girl, Boy, Flower, Bicycle

This girl
Waits at the corner for
This boy
Freewheeling on his bicycle.

She holds
A flower in her hand
A gold flower
In her hands she holds
The sun.
With power between his thighs
The boy

Comes smiling to her
He rides
A bicycle that glitters like
The wind.
This boy this girl
They walk
In step with the wind
Arm in arm
They climb the level street
To where
Laid on the glittering handlebars
The flower
Is round and shining as
The sun.

Heather McPherson

A Money-Bean Tree

My son asks me
for a money-bean tree
and I say when I
find a duchess drawer
that sprouts pink melons
and moonstone eggs
we'll go the rounds
of the Green Witch dens
and offer our spoils
for a money-bean tree—

and we'll live by
the beach and raise
Rhode Island reds
and drink only
goat's milk and honey mead—
and ride white ponies
down to the spit
where we climb Altar Rock
and sit and sit
with lines on our toes

to entice the fish—
and twice a year
we'll light fires
on the sand
and call up the mermaids
and mermen—who'll bring
to our feast: sea
apples and kelp cake
and moon-milk wafers—
and glittering scaly tails—

and some days we'll
wind a fiery thread off
the red-lined clouds
and weave us a basket
to fly out to friends—
or loosen the lightning
and tighten a storm belt
to evacuate dreamers
and refugees from the fumes
of Desperate City—

oh it's just what we
need—a money-bean tree
in the backyard with
peaches and grapes—
we'll rummage the duchess
for moonstone eggs—
maybe package a plea
to the Green Witch direct—
to send us the spell to
make magic belief.

Erick Brenstrum

Wave-runner

for Hugh

At two and a half,
as befits one whose father
twice nearly drowned,
you showed a proper caution

for the sea
and cried for reinforcements
when chased up the beach
by a 3 inch wave.

Now, one year on,
you are a true wave-runner
looping up the wet sand
in a long arc
you swoop down into the foam
shrieking over foot high waves
thrashing up salt water
over your blue shirt

buoyed up by the world
cradled in joy
holding off the trek home
to the triple ritual
of bath books and bed
you circle in the red light of evening
and loop back to the sea
one last time
three more times.

Michael Jackson

from *Fragments*

i

She who was fire to me
and water
and earth
for whom I sang
comes to me now in the wind

I will be healed by music on an empty road
I will fall asleep listening to rivers
I will be warmed by the sun
I will cease to be myself wherever she is

No rain no star no wind will shift for me
no work of the plough no fence
no path

Seven Mysteries

Now write down
the seven mysteries:
why you so young and beautiful should die;
why consciousness prevents
escape into the chestnut branches where
foliage goes soft
with God's vermilion;
why what is said is seldom what was meant;
why men and women work, come home,
cook meals, argue and renew
their vows of silence or revenge;
why we were different;
why there are seven of everything;
why I go on
broken-winded like that horse we saw
on the ridge above Waipatiki
by a bent tree
watching the waves roll in.

Robin Hyde

from *The Beaches*

VI

Close under here, I watched two lovers once,
Which should have been a sin, from what you say:
I'd come to look for prawns, small pale-green ghosts,
Sea-coloured bodies tickling round the pool.
But tide was out then; so I strolled away
And climbed the dunes, to lie here warm, face down,
Watching the swimmers by the jetty-posts
And wrinkling like the bright blue wrinkling bay.
It wasn't long before they came; a fool
Could see they had to kiss; but your pet dunce

Didn't quite know men count on more than that;
And so just lay, patterning the sand.
            And they
Were pale thin people, not often clear of town;

Elastic snapped, when he jerked off her hat;
I heard her arguing, 'Dick, my frock!' But he
Thought she was bread.
I wished her legs were brown,
And mostly, then, stared at the dawdling sea,
Hoping Perry would row me some day in his boat.

Not all the time; and when they'd gone, I went
Down to the hollow place where they had been,
Trickling bed through fingers. But I never meant
To tell the rest, or you, what I had seen;
Though that night, when I came in late for tea,
I hoped you'd see the sandgrains on my coat.

Louis Johnson

Summer Sunday

By the banks of a dried-out creek in the Christmas Hills,
that Sunday in broiling February, we parked the car,
having chosen the backcountry roads for loneliness
rather than bumper-to-bumper progress to beaches;
and under the drying gums with freckles of sun
pocking our bodies, initiated Australia
to our passion for *al fresco* love—launched
our craft on a fragrant forest floor whose heats
intensified our own.
　　　　　　　　The flies were bothersome.
We did not wait long, but took the road
that curved down Big Hill, labelled 1,000 feet,
to the baked township of Yarra Glen, the river
there muddied by the 300 bodies
churning the waters to coffee. You swam
and found it cool, but I would not join you,
some stiffness withholding ability to fling
myself into *any* damn' thing in the name of fun.
I stood on the bank and counted the mounting empties
the local outdoor men heaped against trees
like a kind of memorial to virility.

Don McRae

My Love

My love is rain
Falling on thirsty ground.
My love is light
Shining when all around
The tentacles of night
Imprison and restrain.

My love's a song
Soothing the tired ear.
She is calm
Haven when storms are near,
A healing balm
When pain is fierce and strong.

My love's a cry
Heard in a lonely place.
My love's a flower
Seen on the desert's face
She is a secret bower;
And what am I?

My love is toil
Performed for me and mine.
She is the washing
Hung out upon the line,
And dishes sloshing
And stew put on to boil.

My love's a hand
Held out on pay-day.
She's a reproving judge
Demanding I obey,
An unpaid drudge.
She'd have me understand.

My love's a sigh
Despairing over me (I'll not contest it)
She is a rose
Whose thorns are very near,
A searching nose
That smells my breath for beer;
And what am I? (I think you've guessed it)

Anne French

Boys' Night Out

and they ask each other the questions
none of them has an answer for, like
'Why did she fall for me in the first place
if all she wants to do is change me now?'

> ·   *it's not that simple*

When it's all over is the time the
girls enjoy. They can be best friends then:
sympathise fully (cross your fingers),
analyse everything, and attribute causes.

> *it was never that simple*

But does anyone here know why the white
picket fence is not the answer? Why it makes
us panicky and shrill, thinking we need things
like settling down together, kids, lawns

> *when we could so easily make do with nothing at all*

and why it makes such innocent puzzled
frustrated devious charmers
of them all, drinking and talking their way
through to perfect clarity on the matter?

> *and a full grasp of the easy answer*

Jenny Bornholdt

The Boyfriends

The boyfriends all love you but they don't really know how.

They say it is tragic that you will not be together for the rest of
your lives. You will not be together for the rest of your lives
because they are lone spirits and you are a nice girl,

Because your father is a lawyer and because they like to think they
come from the wrong side of town, they say you will marry a young
lawyer. Someone nice, someone stable, someone able to provide
you with all the things you need and are accustomed to, not a
rogue, not an adventurous spirit like themselves. Not someone
who is destined to the lone life.

They say it will be alright for you. You will be very happy, they can
tell. It will all work out for you. You will find a young lawyer, or a
young lawyer will find you and you will get married and be very happy.
This is what you want, of course.
They say you are made for happiness, anyone can see that.
You will be very happy, you'll see.

They imagine their own sorrow when the day finally comes.
They tell you about this. They imagine seeing you in town with
your new young lawyer. He will have his arm around your
shoulders. You will be looking happy. He will be looking happy.
You will both be looking very happy. They will look on and feel
tragic about it not working out, about the impossibility of the great
love. Because yours is the great love. The true love. Oh yes.
But it cannot work. The great love never works. The true love is
doomed to fail.

You suspect they have seen too many westerns with too many
cowboys riding off into too many sunsets.

In the end of course, you leave him. There isn't really much
choice. He is unhappy. Very unhappy. It is not all that romantic.

When you see him in the street you often cannot speak. You just
look at each other. You both cry a lot in public places. Other
people find this embarrassing and so do you.

He say   please come back.
He says this is the worst thing that has ever happened. And it is.
Please he says. Please.

But you can't. Because it would be going back to leaving him.
You prepared yourself to leave him for years. It took such
a long time.

It took years of listening to him leaving you, knowing that he wouldn't.
All that leaving.
All that is left is the leaving.

Robert Sullivan

from *Community Poems*

4 Hand That Stilled the Water

Went to the DB Onehunga last night. It featured this group
that played Freddy Fender, and the best Samoan lambada this

side of Apia. We drank Double Brown danced and I smiled.
The finer things keep shining through. Reminds me of what Denys

said about Prince Tui Teka, how he was a bigger star
in Rarotonga than David Bowie! Later us guys went back

to the girls' flat. They were singing the gospel.
Something about justice, freedom, and love. In the evening.

In the morning. All over the land. Take your shoes off man,
don't you know you're standing on the ground of paradise?

Evangelism, beautiful women, no more cry.
An ideal system in screwed-up words. Not even those.

My saviour will appear as a love-blaze; you will know
the light. Abba is Jehovah is the glorified King!

Fleur Adcock

An Illustration to Dante

Here are Paolo and Francesca
whirled around in the circle of Hell
clipped serenely together
her dead face raised against his.
I can feel the pressure of his arms
like yours about me, locking.

They float in a sea of whitish blobs—
fire, is it? It could have been
hail, said Ruskin, but Rossetti
'didn't know how to do hail'.
Well, he could do tenderness.
My spine trickles with little white flames.

Tokens

The sheets have been laundered clean
of our joint essence—a compound,
not a mixture; but here are still

your forgotten pipe and tobacco,
your books open on my table,
your voice speaking in my poems.

Bub Bridger

Confession

I'm a little in love with you
Nothing
To cause you embarrassment
Or concern
Just a warm
Skip of the heart
When I see you from
My bus
At your stop

I catch your eye
And give you a wave
And I note
That you are more beautiful
Now than you ever were
And I am a keen
Observer of beauty
Whether it's sunsets
Or music
Or the Mona Lisa
Or birds flying
Or green growing things
Or you

So
How does it feel
My young Adonis to be
Held in such regard

By an elderly lady
On the 24 Express?
Well

Don't knock it
Because it really is
A rare compliment
And you
Only have to respond
With your wide smile
Which is a small price
To pay
For allowing me my glimpse
Of what it used to be
All those years ago
When I was seventeen
And beautiful young men
Smiled
By the dozen

Kevin Ireland

Establishing the Facts

being still quite young
and not wishing to be tricked
I ran my eyes over the small seams

of your skin
checked your blood vessels
twiddled the knobs of your backbone

counted your ribs
took stock of hair and nails
identified such as ears nose throat

vigilantly
I probed on to assure
myself of all your bits and pieces

summed up
their hanging-togetherness
then dismantled them atom by atom

thinking of how
you must have been whirring away
in millions of orbits there beside me

after that
I had to go over you again
and carefully put everything back

then in order
once and for all to be satisfied
I tested out the way you took my strain

until finally
being coupled in a manner
which left nothing whatever in doubt

I could trust a look
into your utterly reliable
eyeballs and confess: darling darling darling

Kendrick Smithyman

Ambush

My life carries on in shadow of terror.
It's a bad habit, living
under threat.
                    In the valley of the shadow
of updating settlement where they've only
lately had their first in living memory,
their first murder since the tribal wars,
we turned off the metal at midday down a track
to the Rotokokahi running over stones.
Every action is a political act.

It happens like that, you are not prepared
for
    bursts of automatic fire *dadadida*,
then a single shot *da* from unseen marksmen
kingfishers, targeting. It happens
like that, as suddenly, a bagatelle and no
one is to blame if fear is all
mixed up with loving. One is seldom
adequate.

Remember that lunch stop by the river?
Kingfishers at their terrorist game and swamp hens
playing up to them like comic strip capers
in and out of shadows. And how childishly
simple I was, loving you loving them, taken over
on the moment while lights jumped and fell
from the bush with another burst of fire
and some ran away down the river.

As though children are ever simple or outgrow
their politics. Mothers tell them,
'Just change your clothes before you go to play.'

Lauris Edmond

Demande de Midi

I wait for you with a reluctant impatience
—it burns, this crucible of an arbitrary
desire; we do not need our youth to teach us
pain, who feel the cramp of habit, know
the slow shaping of the resistant grain.

And it is desperate enough, the act
by which we shall discover the accurate dark
that takes off one by one the customary
authorities of middle life; I fear
the body's cruelly meek discourtesy,

yet listen for your step as though
in the muted clamour of the dusk
there is no other; so eagerly shall I
expose perhaps to folly, cynicism
or neglect the long-protected years.

The evening draws aside to let you through,
I take your hand; like children, as defenceless
and as pure, we guard each other's hesitations.
And should we not so fear to penetrate
the blind and passionate reticence of age?

Iain Sharp

Watching the Motorway by Moonlight

We sit on the viaduct
dangling our toes
in mid-air.
A truckload of turnips
heads towards Auckland
followed by
a carload of nuns
all eating hamburgers
You close your eyes.
Your thoughts become
the night sky
the mist around the moon.
I nudge you gently.

Look, love, at the white moths.
An angel's wing is moulting.

John Summers

Bush Lawyer

Do I love you?
Don't ask so great
a word from me in case
we press beyond the pale
of all I think I am
to find that man
I have not made as yet:
but some floating whale
of lies and hate,
caprice, confusion, lust.

If you must know
I'm only a yo-yo
at Christ's wrist
thrown out by wilful twists
not His, glad to return
to feel His loving touch.
Contrite I hand you this.

By God I'm not free
to nurse a human hate
and fling you from me.
For your dear sake
I long to endure
each dark night
when the nerves crawl
like beetles in the blood,
and mocking I recall
Prometheus and 'literature'.

Don't ask. Don't ask.
Don't take that word,
that pearl of greatest price
I once toyed lightly with
and drop in soured wine
like Cleo, nor emulate
a king's expensive whore
who empties coffers of the state
and starves the poor
to quench a thirst
no lust can ever slake.

But say you love me, do.
Be tender true.
Pretend I am that man
I would be all for you.
Avoid profundities
I might not meet.
Let's kiss your shoulder,
laugh, taste your cheek—
revel in the unpolished rice
about the ramparts,
turn you on: or on
the burning spit of love,
for He that makes the dove,
the lion and the lamb consort
will not forget old Pan.
And I'll forgive you
when you say that's typical,
and spoken like a man.

R.A.K. Mason

Thigh to Thigh

Thigh to thigh and lip to lip
    in the long grass we lie
      the cup brims high but we dare not sip

Girl don't you think that we were meant
    to take it and drink
      to blend and sink back in drowsed content?

But the seconds pass the moment's gone
    and the rustling grass
      breathes a dead mass and an orison

And two night birds toll from a star-lit bough
    dirge-voiced the waves roll
      as though a soul were passing now.

Elizabeth Smither

St Paul's Kind of Love

How does one preserve oneself for it
The kind of gentle not-puffed-up
Love which endlessly bears
But never swells like a camel
With fat resentment?
Was St Paul thinking of a place
Somewhere behind women's hats
Where women could take them off
And let their hair stream
In a safe bedroom light?
Did the crusty saint
Really have a vision
Of two days' delight?

Sarah Quigley

Anglo-Indian Summer

sitting outside
the woodstock arms
you trap moody

wasps in empty
beer glasses. i tidy
crisp packets

into 8s 16s
or 32s and fold myself
away from you.

swedish girls
interpret the air
between us

and stay away
because infidelity
has a sting

in any language.

Denis Glover

I'm an Odd Fish

I'm an Odd Fish
A No-Hoper:
Among Men a Snapper,
Among Women
A Groper.

The Two Flowers

To man or woman I say
It's foolish to think
It's roses or lilies all the way,
Roses blood-red, lilies that stink.
Take life with both hands,
Take dark blood, take foul,
Then use a towel.

Michael Harlow

Only on the White

In the tattoo parlour at Easter
there is an arrangement in which everything
takes place; love is happening at once.
You imagine you begin life as a heliotrope;
everyone begins to take off their clothes,
shake small bells at ankle, at wrist.
Oh this high holiday of the body, we touch
each other under shivers of light;
the songs we sing.

At the street-window there are clouds
of elderly gentlemen in coloured clothes;
they are in urgent need of information,
and the 'lost noises of the sun'.
When the word is passed round, flowers
fly through the air; there are psalms
growing out of the piano: for Lent
the tattooed Lady plays only on the white.

Bob Orr

Signatures

Dawn unpinned
the stars
that had sheeted
the night
down over us.

A lopsided tree
leant bright
against our window.
A feathering of leaves
whispered like the sea
of coasts kept only
in memory.

Your eyelids
closed estuaries
of dream.

Your hair rained
in the half dark room.
My veins guttered into
blue oceans.

Outside
the looped flight
of pigeons stitched
the streets

to the sky.

Kathleen Gallagher

I Love You Annie

'I love you Annie'
she looked at him laughing
'you're a taxicab driver
I come from the mountains
you're a taxicab drive

and I can't sing here
you breathe like a city
I sing like the mountains'
'but I love you Annie'
he saw the snow in her eyes

Jenny Bornholdt

In Love

This is a piece
to fit.
It is the piece
about her being
in love.
It should belong between the
piece of her before being
in love and the piece
of her after being
in love.
Instead it covers
everything.
The heart has no corners
and is stretched
to its limit.

James K. Baxter

At the Fox Glacier Hotel

One kind of love, a Tourist Bureau print
Of the Alps reflected in Lake Matheson

(Turned upside down it would look the same)
Smiles in the dining room, a lovely mirror

For any middle-aged Narcissus to drown in—
I'm peculiar; I don't want to fall upwards

Into the sky! Now, as the red-eyed tough
West Coast beer-drinkers climb into their trucks

And roar off between colonnades
Of mossed rimu, I sit for a while in the lounge

In front of a fire of end planks
And wait for bedtime with my wife and son,

Thinking about the huge ice torrent moving
Over bluffs and bowls of rock (some other

Kind of love) at the top of the valley—
How it might crack our public looking-glass

If it came down to us, jumping
A century in twenty minutes,

So that we saw, out of the same window
Upstairs where my underpants are hanging to dry,

Suddenly—no, not ourselves
Reflected, or a yellow petrol hoarding,

But the other love, yearning over our roofs
Black pinnacles and fangs of toppling ice.

Lauris Edmond

A Reckoning

You were my friend, accomplice in
the copious plotting parents are a party to;
through centuries of jovial boredom
on the beach we stuck it out together

then separately awake hallucinated
over teenage accidents in cars, until
a door at last breathed out and cracks
of guilty silence shot us dead asleep.

Our fears kept us close; pride too,
and the small events' unmerciful momentum.
It was a walled garden, safe to quarrel in,
love coming down on us reliably as rain.

We were its keepers, so intent we did not see
the change of sky, the gradual departures
—then there was just a man, a woman
slamming some old gate on a quiet plot

ill-tempered without learnt weather
and the rule of law. Who were
the guardians then, and who, despite
that virtuous authority, the guarded?

Alan Riach

Necessity of Listening

(for John Purser)

Love makes belief in miracles,
and future brings its own time, not the past's
predictions. You're right enough,
John: we should be content, contented.

Today, your new boat rests
in chuckling water, moored near Glasgow.
Soon you will take her to Skye.
Your hand will rest and move upon the tiller.

Tonight, my wife: her hand upon my arm
now knows no source for its resting;
her sleeping smile is unknowing as I am;
her comfort content is my own, her husband.

Fleur Adcock

Afterwards

We weave haunted circles about each other,
advance and retreat in turn, like witchdoctors
before a fetish. Yes, you are right to fear
me now, and I you. But love, this ritual

will exhaust us. Come closer. Listen. Be brave.
I am going to talk to you quietly
as sometimes, in the long past (you remember?),
we made love. Let us be intent, and still. Still.
There are ways of approaching it. This is one:
this gentle talk, with no pause for suspicion,
no hesitation, because you do not know
the thing is upon you, until it has come—
now, and you did not even hear it.
                                        Silence
is what I am trying to achieve for us.
A nothingness, a non-relatedness, this
unknowing into which we are sliding now
together: this will have to be our kingdom.

Rain is falling. Listen to the gentle rain.

Fleur Adcock

Happy Ending

After they had not made love
she pulled the sheet up over her eyes
until he was buttoning his shirt:
not shyness for their bodies—those
they had willingly displayed—but a frail
endeavour to apologise.

Later, though, drawn together by
a distaste for such 'untidy ends'
they agreed to meet again; whereupon
they giggled, reminisced, held hands
as though what they had made was love—
and not that happier outcome, friends.

Fiona Kidman

Earthquake Weather

For three days now, the air
has been quiet and still.
Yesterday, a vase walked across
the mantelpiece. A friend and I
have traced the fault line
along a map. It is very close.
There is neither sun, nor yet rain,
and the wind has departed too.
The crickets have stopped singing
and the children's' quarrels grown bitter.
We wait, sealed in this
grey vacuum.

And when we went to bed
last night, the moon slanted
between the curtains (yes,
we still have a moon),
catching your white smile
in a dazzling glitter. We
who have known rage and lust,
regrets and promises, have come
to understand love. I was afraid
that you were about to devour me.
I wish this weather
would break soon.

Brian Turner

Wife

You have put out the light.
The radio speaks to us, distantly, from the front room.
Your hair falls over your tragic face:
Your eyes are full of tears.
You move closer
And your breathing keeps pace with mine.
I lower my head, listen
To the beating of your heart
And the muffled, far-off roar of the sea.

Lauris Edmond

Epithalamion

for L.E.R.

Wife, woman, hausfrau, female companion
you are rightly summoned again
to the careful ceremony. But you know,
you never left off being married
as you went on guarding your supplies
(ripening figs, soup stock, pears
to be bottled) with a gentle managing tact
somehow avoiding the crowd of waiting
ambitions while you nourished the cells
of the house—a grandchild's teddy bear
the failing lasiandra bushes . . .

wife, wif, woman, let me redefine the notion
stand it before me, observe
the natural wave of its greying hair
the unclamorous refrain of the voice
and the confident smell of a cleaned kitchen
and labelled jars glinting, a whiff
of cut grass at the window—

yes the wife in you, widowed, kept up
its daily preparation of house room
for the heart, stayed mysteriously content
with the ancient humilities
a lit fire, a boiling kettle
the deep solace of bread.

Alistair Te Ariki Campbell

To My Grandson Oliver Maireriki Aged One Day

Fierce little warrior,
What are you dreaming of
In your pre-dawn sleep?
The ancestral carver

Who jealously preserves
The stern family likeness
Has carved your small face
From obsidian, denting
The bridge of the nose
So that you grimly frown
As if bracing yourself
To wake up in a world
Far removed from the warm
Maternal waters of Tongareva
Where you had waited
All these years to be born,
Moulded in the spirit
Of the last anointed *ariki*
Whose proud name you bear.
Dearest blood of the land,
The wonder of your parents,
Elizabeth and Gregory,
Through whom our ancestors
Express their brooding care,
What more can I wish you than
The fulfilment of your dreams,
Love and peace of mind
And the world to enjoy?

Fiona Farrell

Jigsaw

In a corner of their bedroom
under dust they
keep their jigsaw.

On wet evenings they
reassemble the patterns
of summer.

Trees and the smell of mushrooms
twigs in her mouth
sweating grass
spotted sheets

babies and cats and a red carpet
a bay and the wipers going
one　　　　　　　two
one　　　　　　　two.

But she keeps some pieces
tucked among her hankies

and he has a bit of the sky
locked away
in a small drawer.

Michele Leggott

Keeping Warm

you there at
the long end
of my arm

drive me to
work & back
over the bridge

to distraction
icecreams in
the wind or

moon on the
beach: *them*
dauphins

berserk about
us on their
offshore roads

razzle dazzle
moonlight
climb up the

near side of
heaven's cloudy
smile: this is

heaven & you
in it following
la vie dansante

warm rowdy
voice reading
to the kids

draped word
perfect about
you doing

equal parts
charm & need
for me looking

on decoding
nuance (oh
clouds) the house

needs a paint
the Saturday
skilsaws howl

into September
& cups of tea
punctuate the

hard questions
: there was a
moment when

that look in
your eye closed
all distances

ka-boom as
the poets say
dreamily

two people
get together
like *spring*

and *moon*
time & place
fold around

them: yes
there's specific
moonlight and

a curve in
the road where
it takes your

breath away
this is local
right here up

close & it's
your bridge to
where I stand

laughing at
it already
written in

big glittering
letters: let's
go out there

and do the poem

Eileen Duggan

The Tides Run Up the Wairau

The tides run up the Wairau
That fights against their flow.
My heart and it together
Are running salt and snow.

For though I cannot love you,
Yet, heavy, deep, and far,
Your tide of love comes swinging,
Too swift for me to bar.

Some thought of you must linger,
A salt of pain in me,
For oh what running river
Can stand against the sea?

Ruth Gilbert

Green Hammock, White Magnolia Tree

(F.M.G.)

They cannot speak who have no words to say.
If, in my songs, I have not sung of you
It is because I could not find a way.

How in the grace-note of a phrase convey
Such melody, such cadence as we knew?
They cannot speak who have no words to say.

What metaphor, what image dare obey
Love's first command, the praise that is your due?
And though I seek, I have not found a way.

It is the past, the memories that betray,
The backward look, the introspective view,
They cannot speak who have no words to say.

Green hammock, white magnolia, yesterday,
The haunted bough, the great flowers choked with dew—
Love, it is here words lost and lose their way.

Is there no homage that my heart can pay?
You were the sun in whose clear light we grew,
But it is vain; I have not found a way.
They cannot speak who have no words to say.

Tony Beyer

Losing You

that night we drove to the airport
bracken threatening the headlights
elton john's *funeral for a friend*
on the cassette player
                    all your props
arranged to perfection in the storming dark

the terminal lounge was full
of fragmentary americans delayed
by skies indifferent to travellers
and you by the set of your mouth
familiar from childhood
signalled your choice of joining them

in my memory now our bare hands
clasp and part with a tearing sound
and not one word we said
above the engines' yell and intercom
and cackle of baggage carts remains
to settle me for brotherhood across
an ocean wider than my reach
or narrow inward seas of separateness

earthbound and tribal I watched
your flight recede into an eye fault
over the mud flats
thinking how much of love
is what we have managed poorly
but enjoyed
        and then small things
like the ride home
and one or two brief errands on the way

Bill Sewell

Bread and Wine

These are the fundamentals:
   you and I, an avocado pear
with vinaigrette (all tanginess
   and texture), a dry white,
a whole evening ahead of us,
   and a night.

How one sense usurps another:
   we devour also with our
eyes, gazing across the table

to share the flavour. While
our tongues caress each spoonful,
 scooped frugally out.

I know there are mechanisms
 murmuring here, to do with
continuity, with survival. But
 they don't show their workings
tonight. Tonight, we're simply,
 selfishly alive.

And we don't need a priest
 to make our offering, nor
a congregation in which to lose
 ourselves. We offer, we lose
ourselves to one another, assisted
 by an avocado.

Meg Campbell

Sea Creatures

Under the sea
are the whale noises;
above the sea
the noise of doves.
Under the sea,
or above the sea,
I am in your arms.
Under the bed
lies the dog Nanook.
He hears the whales,
the doves, and sighs,
'These humans!' But we
are sea creatures,
you and I.

C.K. Stead

from *From the Clodian Songbook*

2

Clodia's pigeon pair
                    one on egg-guard
the other at large
or roosting above tomatoes
heavy with their siftings—

          she likes the hard peck
they give her fingers

                    she likes their talk
of rolled oats
under the awning.

Ignoring my parallel season
        she ripens in her deck chair
            eating the stained fruit.

I too like that tang on the tongue
                softness of feather
pain of the sharp peck.

Hone Tuwhare

Love Pome

How beautifully
your fingers interlock: how
decorously decorative.
Must you pick your nose like that?

But how uncommonly comely.

How uncrucially crucial:
shuddering balls! Woman
you unsex me farting glib and
gustily.

O, but how utterly homely.

Iain Sharp

The Constitution

Elizabeth lies beside me.
She'd like a story, she says,
a lullaby, an anecdote.
She wants a few words
to prove our connection.

I ransack my brain
for some delectable phrase
to describe the way she breathes,
the way her eyes are,
but even with a lure
finer than a plankton net,
there's nothing,
nothing I can capture.

I believe the love that lasts
has little need of language.
It gathers as slowly,
as inexorably,
as the seeping of stalactites
to form an underground lake
in limestone country.

I think of such a lake.
I lie a long while in silence
staring at the blank ceiling
while Elizabeth grows impatient.
She coughs. She taps my shoulder.
At last, defeated, I say:
Imagine how small atoms are,
yet they constitute all matter.

Bill Manhire

Children

The likelihood is
the children will die
without you to help them do it.
It will be spring,
the light on the water,
or not.

And though at present
they live together
they will not die together.
They will die one by one
and not think to call you:
they will be old

and you will be gone.
It will be spring,
or not. They may be crossing
the road,
not looking left,
not looking right,

or may simply be afloat at evening
like clouds unable
to make repairs. That
one talks too much, that one
hardly at all: and they both enjoy
the light on the water

John Barr

The Bachelor's Resolve

'I wish I had married,'
    Quo' bachelor John,
As he sat himsel' down
    Wi' a sigh and a moan;

'I wish I had married,
  Before 'twas too late,
For I'm noo an auld Batch,
  That's a fact true as fate.

'I wish I had married
  When I had my youth,
Noo nane will tak' me,
  That's a plain gospel truth;
The day has gone by,'
  And he heavily groaned,
'I'm noo an auld Batch
  In the slough o' despond.

'I thocht to mysel',
  If I e'er took a wife,
That I ne'er would grow rich
  A' the days o' my life;
But what o' my wealth,
  Or wha cares for me,
Unless when they wish
  For the day that I'll dee?

'I wash my ain sarks,
  And I darn my ain hose,
I make my ain kale,
  And I make my ain brose;
I toil like a nigger
  Wi' grub, hoe, or spade,
And when it gets dark
  I crawl off to my bed.

'When I see honest men
  Wi' their wives by their side,
When I see decent lads
  At the kirk wi' their bride,
I hang doon my head
  As I slip hame alane,
To my cheerless, my wifeless,
  My cauldrife hearthstane.

'By jingo,' quo' John,
  'I will yet try my luck,
There's aulder than me
  That young Cupid has struck;

Come weal, or come woe,
   I will stand this nae mair,
There are nae fools like auld fools,
   The deevil may care.

'I'll get a new suit
   O' the true Wilkie cut,
I'll shave my lang beard,
   And I'll wash off the smut;
Then I'll doon to young Nancy,
   Sae trig and sae braw,
If she'll tak' me, she'll get me,
   My cash, kye, and a'.'

Jenny Bornholdt

Wedding Song

Now you are married
try to love the world
as much as you love
each other. Greet it as your husband,
wife. Love it with all your
might as you sleep
breathing against its back.

Love the world, when, late at night,
you come home to find snails
stuck to the side of the house
like decoration.

Love your neighbours.
The red berries on their trampoline
their green wheelbarrow.

Love the man walking on
water, the man up a
mast. Love the light moving
across the *Island Princess*.

Love your grandmother when she tells you
her hair is three-quarters 'café au lait'.

Try to love the world, even when you discover
there is no such thing as *The Author*
any more.

Love the world, praise
god, even, when your aerobics instructor
is silent.

Try very hard to love
your mailman, even though he regularly
delivers you Benedicto Clemente's mail.

Love the weta you find on the path,
injured by alteration.

Love the tired men, the burnt
house, the handlebars of light
on the ceiling.

Love the man on the bus who says
it all amounts to a fishing rod
or a light bulb.

Love the world of the garden.
The keyhole of bright green grass
where the stubborn palm
used to be,
bees so drunk on ginger flowers
that they think the hose water
is rain   your hair tangled in
heartsease.   Love the way,
when you come inside,
insects find their way out
from the temporary rooms of
your clothes.

Part 4

Time slipped through our fingers

Bernadette Hall

Duck

there's a duck on the road
its head sticking out of the shiny dark
twisting like a tap turned on turned off

it's hurt, it's stuck
on the thin white line that divides
four lanes of manic traffic

why did the duck cross the road?
because she thought she had to
because her mother had done it before
because she didn't think
because she didn't think she had to think
because she was hungry

onoff onoff onoff

consider for a moment
the domestic situation of the duck:
the rough nip on the neck the bluster
the headshove under water
the fluster and wing flap indignant
the flash of an indigo armband

why did she fall for it this time?
the fat wibble wobble of a batty criss cross trundle
on the Main South Road, ten little Speights babies
left tweedling on the thick brown skin of the river
she didn't know / oh yes she did
oh no she didn't / too right she did
she knew damned well and she should have known better

onoff onoff onoff

someone's got to do something
oh yeah! she's made her bed and now she'll have to lie in it
you'd be far better off to whack her on the head
and put her out of her misery
just how much can you afford to invest in a duck anyway?

this is a classic film noir
one of us is the femme fatale
one is the chap's best friend
I just wish I could remember the ending!

I'm a gymnast on a narrow beam
I ride the slipstream of hot metal
it's wet, the road is slippery
people are in a hurry to get home
I'm a collapsing Z

I grab the duck

> the twiggy cretonne feathers scissorslip
> a bit I dig harder into her hot gut the way
> I would if I was stuffing her before basting

I wrench her off the road

> dumb demure dappling   her neck wobbling
> away from me   her open beak   her dribble

I hold up the duck like a trophy

WOMAN KILLED IN RUSH HOUR TRAFFIC
SHE WAS TAKING HER LIFE IN HER HANDS
SHE WAS HOLDING A DUCK IN HER HANDS
SHE WAS OLD ENOUGH TO KNOW BETTER

all the way home I crash the gears crying
and I rush into the house to get a blanket
and the others say what's wrong
and I say I've got a runover duck in the car
and I need a blanket and they all start to laugh
and make helpful suggestions like

it won't make any difference
I've got more to worry about than a bloody duck
it'll be dead by now anyway and there's no room
left in the garden to bury things, god almighty,
we've already got two dogs, three mice, five goldfish
and the rabbit buried there, what more do you want?

and they're right of course
when I go out to bring her in
she's dead

aue! aue! what will I do with you, *my own aisling*?

Queen of Spades in a brown tweed coat,
rock skimmer in scungy water, corky decoy,
topsy turvy lady of dibble and dabble, mud shoveller,
funny puddler, silly quack quack

Robin Healey

Night Kitchen

In the dream she turns my head
in her small hands so gently
to kiss her dark mouth,
we are in a dark kitchen, I think,
the black panes reflect us,
then it is bone, elastic on bone,
nothing there.

It stays with me all the fractious day,
somebody observes the over forties
become pillars of the community.
I visit a friend grey with illness,
pitiless, nothing fits, a mouthful of dust.

Walking it off tonight
past the dark windows of white painted houses,
wooden nightgowns caught in flight,
the moon is a deep gold crescent
a star poised above it.

In the dream she turned my head
so gently, drew me in with such small hands,
I was so pleased by the touch
of her softly pleated red mouth
in that dark. The moon and a star
are poised, just poised in the huge cold.

Sam Hunt

Stabat Mater

My mother called my father 'Mr Hunt'
For the first few years of married life.
I learned this from a book she had inscribed:
'To dear Mr Hunt, from his loving wife.'

She was embarrassed when I asked her why
But later on explained how hard it had been
To call him any other name at first, when he—
Her father's elder—made her seem so small.

Now in a different way, still like a girl,
She calls my father every other sort of name;
And guiding him as he roams old age
Sometimes turns to me as if it were a game . . .

That once I stand up straight, I too must learn
To walk away and know there's no return.

David Howard

from *The Last Word*

3

Honeymooning at Pines Beach,
we'd lie spellbound by a spider's craft.
While bumblebees got drunk
on dandelion wine
it would hide behind a petal, sensing
their secret ambition was to suck
the nipple-pink rose
it had built its home and hopes on . . .

Alone, I thread berries onto a briar stem
then count my 'blessings'
on this god-forsaken rosary. I should settle
for wine and song: my woman
sleeps in a winding sheet
the spider might have woven.

Kevin Ireland

A Way of Sorrow

for James K. Baxter

when quite by chance
I heard that you were dead
I did not weep
or talk at length or write
but read the poem you sent
then went back to my love
and climbed her stairs
and in her light-dark bed
I lay down bare
beneath her weight
and while she gripped
with all her strength
the tearless speechless nameless
grief in me I stared
into her shroud-white face
and the stark black border
of her hair

Sam Hunt

August Steam

The lake made no sense early on:
driving down a slipway straight
two truant kids in a big V8
parking in a rain storm
huddled in beside the lake.

It made no sense then early on:
it wasn't till much later
we understood things better
nothing could go wrong—
you said let's drive forever.

We could only return:
the sulphur city drenched
steaming after rain: so ditched
the faithful love machine
made in for a dressing shed.

Undressed each other in turn:
I never thought I'd ever
be your winter hot-pool lover
until I was right then.
Some things are never over.

Vivienne Plumb

Women Often Dream of Flying

At one o'clock
she dreams of flying over
clouds, choppy frozen
lakes or ploughed blue fields.
Patterns emerge, rivers,
valleys and volcanoes.

Her skull tingles.

In the distance
the sun sinks, leaving a bright rind
on the horizon. The sky
tumbles down and touches cloud, melting
into one new chemistry equation.

She's flying
and she thinks she's in love.

She wakes, finds she's
landed on gorse, a great
spread of it. This is her life now,
thorns and the hard yellow of old
yolks. This is a type of love.

Louis Johnson

Statistics

The survey showed, that on this particular night,
of 2020 couples polled, throughout the city
there were 1714 men who stood in their garages
debating whether to get back into the car and drive
off. For ever. Of these, 1608 had a plan of somewhere
to go or had already become involved with a mistress
or an adulterous relationship with a friend's
wife. Of these, 110 were convinced their wives
were already having it off with the friend. Twelve
thought that a fair exchange. One said he thought
they deserved each other. Their mean average age
was 44. The average wife was two years shorter.
Most believed they could still better themselves: twelve
didn't care. One had given up hope. But didn't go.
Instead, he went into the house, manoeuvringly,
opened the door and shoved his spouse headfirst
down the cellar steps where for once she lay quiet
and unprotesting. He answered the door, filled in the survey,
then filled the bath and cut his throat with an old
steelblade razor that had belonged to grandfather.
Most polled said they felt desperate but not enough
to kill. Most had mortgages and felt uncertain
of all their choices—partners, jobs, the names
of the children, the house and furniture; especially
the wall decorations and pictures. Nearly half
had an original painting on the wall. Twenty-seven
had bought or read a volume of poems in the past year.
It appears the anarchy of art has little to do with
their drive to destruction, their disaffection, and desperate
disappointment with society. All felt cheated. All
lit up when asked if they thought the game was worth
the candle. One said he always did it by torchlight.
Which reminded him of his outdoor interests in youth.
Most owned, or wanted to own, a waterbed.

Of the wives, 973 thought it was ownership of the children
that kept the men coming home. Most of them did it late.
The Kinsey average of three times a week for their class,
education and financial status seemed much too much.
But 723 thought they might manage more with a lover;

lamented the high cost of baby-sitters: 927 favoured return
to the single bed but preferred the waterbed with its cooling
rhythms for entertaining the lover. A drop in the price
of analgesics was recommended by most. One wife wanted
more so much it was the wanting gave her the headaches:
she'd taken two whole bottles once and ended in Ward 10
fellating a stomach-pump: 430 had scars on both wrists.
One hundred and seventy-three had separate careers: two
worked with their spouses in home industries. Most thought
sterilization of the male after the first 2.2 children would
be the best preservative of the married estate: it might
eliminate competition, allow the parents to concentrate
on governing kids. Most identified their mates with one
animal or another—rats and snakes being the most favoured.
Seventy-two percent had their own car: three knew
how to change a wheel or mend a puncture. Most
shared, or wanted to share, a waterbed.

The conclusions we draw are that marriage, in our time,
is under serious pressure. Allowance is made
for a three-percent margin of error in the findings.
There is a much higher failure-rate in marriage itself.
The poll was sponsored by Mobile Pneumatic Bliss—
makers of Fly United waterbeds.

Fiona Kidman

from *Wakeful Nights*

3

Leigh, North Auckland the Jolly
Fisherman's Lodge, approached
from the wharves over slatted
wooden bridges,   suitcases
in hand.   Your letter arrived
for my birthday 1960:
'surprise surprise two letters
from me and none from you, send
me a telegram when you
decide.' All I did was read

all week watching the spinifex
turn over on the sand. Only
when the distant lights of boats shone
through the shadow of the navy
sea burning beyond the granite
cliffs, the haunted clay,
was it cool enough to consider
your proposal;
                        in the end
I said yes, a strange
place to choose a life.

4

In the dark the children's faces
like magnolia flowers on the pillows.
Whose turn to chase the milkman's
night delivery down the frosty road
the forgotten bottles clanking
against our dressing gowns? Those
children drank 8 pints a day.

5

These wakeful nights went hand
in hand with grit, mad laughter
and tears; they were bodies turning
left to right right to left
against the gaunt, the red-eyed
dream. We listened to the winds
that sweep across
        Te Whanganui a Tara,
their muttered *kiss gasp kiss*
at the window pane, as we sought
each other's bones.   Instead
of resting, we tore the blankets
from side to side, avenging
late parties, nightmares, ordinary deceits.
Oh, in the end, we said
                        enough.

6

As the last light star
dissolves above the sea, you
place the white cup beside
the bed, love so various
has become kind: 'how did
            you sleep?' the ritual
enquiry;

                  'not badly'
I tell you,
      remembering
   one thought leading
to the next as the Judas
sheep leads its brothers up
the slaughterhouse ramp and
slips away, words ever
treacherous; the notebooks
go on filling night
            by lighted night,
those hours at last are friends.

   Do not think me changed, my
fabled fault and virtue to
love persistently, nothing
changes that.   I have simply
learned to guard the word
beyond the powerful dark;
            the sun fans along the hill
tops, I watch the bay, the sky
the heavy heavy languor
of the green curtain lifting.

Michael Jackson

Parentage

Were we ordered to play in this garden
or tempted out in the bright
disintegrating autumn light
by a blackbird flying
across the frosted lawn?

All morning I thought I heard them
arguing beyond the wide verandah
while the warped boards where
I had driven splinters into my hands
trembled with the rough words.

Was it my father, and the other,
was it her,
was it her with a fur-lined coat who
would lean and smother me each night
beside the darkened stair,

Pretend to bite my father's ear off,
laugh and spin, showering kisses
and spilling her pink gin?
                    It was not my mother.
And my father, was it really him?

Leonard Lambert

The Lovers at Sixty

Loyal to the image
they hold of one another,
the old young dog
& his innuendo whore
the lovers at sixty.

At home the cupboards
are packed with wounding fact,
convictions of every possible
human failing hang
on numbered nails.

But superbly saved
by the cued aside
this show enters its
45th fantastic year
as to soft applause
they enter bow perform,
that lovely waltzing pair
the lovers at sixty.

Iain Lonie

A Postcard of Cornwall

The harbour wall, sunlight on the water
the blue boats, and the bookshop of a lost language—
I can feel you taking it all.

Look, already the colours fade in the mind:
only the name stays to signify a place
where two made love in the deep grass of June.

Were they really ourselves? Gently, persistently
I feel you working at it, working it all away
under the bright surface that divides our elements.

Soon, if you go on like this
I shall have nothing left. Take it, then:
or anything that helps.

Your needs are unimaginable. The sun-
filled estuary, widening to the sea—
take it all. Take me.

Kendrick Smithyman

Could You Once Regain

Girl, could you once regain
that pitiless mask!
                It is drawn
through the flesh's suffering
from your inmost tranquil bone,
when, shaken by love you lie
purged of the weights of a day,
your face unbelievably pure
as though bone lit with clarity,
transparency fired by the act
of love to possess your feature
and sharpen out of its firing
some other disguised nature.

If you held that purity
of your body, then, in repose,
where knowledge had seemed to be
self-knowing, self-aware—
                              I propose
a chaos. For should you go out
in the bitter livid street,
the young would be disgraced, bent
men be momently straight,
the huddled world raise a shout
for the face not seen since the day
when a wall and a city went down
and the Trojan suffered the clown
to stare on her pride.

                              I pray
again to be snared by that light
floods from your face when love
has shaken us through and world
is most perfectly perceived
by the afterglow, as the light
dies back to the tranquil bone,
and, commingling, we may stretch
and companionably yawn,
resuming the suffering flesh
by which we are daily grieved.

Bernadette Hall

Amica

for Joanna

The house is a reliquary
of insects, flowers & fingernails
& this is rare, Amica, that you assume
with your Etruscan air its essence;
lying on the hill arch of your arm;
on a sarcophagus. Someone is whistling
in the kitchen, laying down new territory

with aluminium brightness. All the windows
are open. Ivory tides wash out, wash in
& you sing the mysteries: that love
is a gift; that nothing is ever lost;
that death is the centre of a long life.

Bob Orr

Sugar Boat

The black sugar boat
across the bay
beneath the chains of Chelsea—
we saw it from the other side of town
moored up by the refinery. We were sitting
on the hard steps of a jetty in Herne Bay. The waves
kept coming in—a yellow crust
of cool volcanic moon
flew up above the
city.
  We were close
to breaking up. We could only see ourselves
through images. The jetty was adrift
in jagged light. A dark wind was blowing in on us.
I saw you as I never had before . . . as you
swam slowly towards your freedom
as the phosphorescent sea
became the tail of a mermaid
between your feet
as I kept turning
& as a black sugar boat
     across the bay was burning.

W.H. Oliver

A *Performance of* Death and the Maiden

On a sultry evening, in the college hall,
Young men and women gather to hear the music
Our deathwards Schubert wrote about a girl,
Her battle with death, his and her subtle tricks.
She was, of women, silly, splendid and blind;
She thought to break the chain original sin
Forged of men mating—as if forgoing the risk
Were not the strongest link within that chain
And love the tenderest loosener she'd find.

Sable-cloaked youths, hot from the road and the river,
Lead in their maidens, sunbaked and brownarmed,
Hinting at dispositions too delicate to be harmed,
Teetering strollers on the high taut wire
Poised between novice and deliberate performer,
Hesitant, flaunting, cold in their colours of fire.
From flaming chestnut walks and buttercup fields,
From the Thames carefully carrying fastidious cargoes
Stretched on her boats, slack beneath masculine clouds,
They enter the oppressive shadows of wall and window.

The players call to battle, and follow the wavering fight.
Then men in black grow tall with the power of him
Who tricked the subtle maiden with his grin.
The sunny river girls see night erect
And stark as graveyards stilt across the room.
The music ends, too frantic. Whom do they acclaim?
The cloaked deceiver or that stringent girl?
They walk away to their separate narrow cots
Shaken with prodigal feats they'll need to learn:
For all round flesh must die if left unslain.

Alistair Te Ariki Campbell

Why Don't You Talk to Me?

Why do I post my love letters
in a hollow log?
Why put my lips to a knothole in a tree
and whisper your name?

The spiders spread their nets
and catch the sun,
and by my foot in the dry grass
ants rebuild a broken city.

Butterflies pair in the wind,
and the yellow bee,
his holsters packed with bread,
rides the blue air like a drunken cowboy.

More and more I find myself
talking to the sea.
I am alone with my footsteps.
I watch the tide recede
and I am left with miles of shining sand.

Why don't you talk to me?

Louis Johnson

Dirge

We built our love up like a work of art,
Increasing and subtracting as we came
First through the birth-world of redoubled Spring
And afterwards through flame.

But when the hell of the attendant smoke
Burst through the chemistry of you and I,
We were the victims of each other's hands
Not knowing how or why.

We consumed love at that first brief encounter,
And having nothing, on each other turned
With hands of hate to tear the other up
To see if love still burned.

Ruth Gilbert

Rachel

Black night without, and blacker night within,
Night we had dreamed both bountiful and wise,
Night that spurned Rachel, smiled on Leah's sin
And willed a blindness on my lover's eyes.

There were no stars, and clouds upon the moon
Darkened the vine-yards; restively astir
Winds cried among the olive-boughs too soon
And Leah spoke, and Jacob answered her . . .

He came in singing, singing from the feast,
Singing our love and the long years fulfilled,
Singing my beauty, and the dark increased
And anguish walked until his song was stilled . . .

My love, my love, had you not wit to guess
Another mouth than mine beneath your own?
Had Leah's hands no alien tenderness,
Her voice no strange, no unfamiliar tone?

I can forgive you everything but this—
Laban and Leah struck no keener blow—
One stole my bridal, one my marriage kiss,
But you were blind, and slept, and did not know.

Bill Manhire

My Sunshine

He sings you are my sunshine
and the skies are grey, she tries
to make him happy, things
just turn out that way.

She'll never know
how much he loves her
and yet he loves her so much
he might lay down his old guitar
and walk her home, musician
singing with the voice alone.

Oh love is sweet and love is all, it's
evening and the purple shadows fall
about the baby and the toddler
on the bed. It's true he loves her
but he should have told her,
he should have, should have said.

Foolish evening, boy with a foolish head.
He sighs like a flower above his instrument
and his sticky fingers stick. He fumbles
a simple chord progression,
then stares at the neck.
He never seems to learn his lesson.

Here comes the rain. Oh if she were only
sweet sixteen and running from the room again,
and if he were a blackbird
he would whistle and sing
and he'd something
something something something.

Donald McDonald

Time

Upon the benchy hillside
Where hoggets love to lie,
With noses pointed to the wind
And half-closed eye,
I walked alone on Sundays,
And wished my love was nigh.
For oh! the hours went slower
Than the moon goes in the sky.

Upon the benchy hillside
Raked with wind and sun,
Where the grey hawk hovers
And little rabbits run,

My love and I did linger
A few short hours;
But time slipped through our fingers,
As the wind slips through the flowers!

Martha Morseth

Broken Porcelain

The roundness of the cup
    fits my stone hands
The hot tea warms
    my fingers
The morning light is fragile,
    like the delicate pattern
    of blue on white porcelain.

The willows bend lightly, stroking
the bridge, dip their angular
fingers to touch the lovers.
He bends to kiss her gently,
she is brave, he promises to write.

You see a crack, a miniscule spider
    thread, reaching from
    the bottom to the lip.
You say it harbours disease, even
    now the microbes are
    amassing battalions to
    join the surge of tea
    to my lips.

I think of that summer day beside
the Taieri. The willows touched the
black water, the air breathed the scent
of spring, I promised to stay forever.

We sit together in the kitchen
You break the cup
    wrap it in paper
        throw it away.
Now we are safe, you say.

Michele Leggott

Dear Heart

dear heart it was a coast road
long past lilac time and well out of town
                                        the sea out of sight   and driving north
                                        in the far south the radio swelled
                        nostalgia
                        and I want you to know
                                                that I remember it all   the time
        it was 'just' part of your afternoon repertoire
        a dance-floor pick-up
                        kept on at you all those years   the romance the real
                        life dance we were brought in to share
        the sun and the son
        you were making it true with a late-fifties step
                                                up the coast   into heaven
                        and some memorable parties
                        fishing trips
                                carnivals
                                        a dog   a truck   a baby sister
                a walk to the swing bridge
        and back
                and more . . .

                then it was moving into town   settling
                down and later the piano
                                        you were picking out Mancini arrangements
Nat King Cole My Fair Lady and the theme
from Mondo Cane
                you sang them into the woodwork
                and when it really was
                                a table for one and a single rose
                                that hard lost time
        I heard Errol Garner play I only
        have eyes for you in a winter house   dancing
                                        with knots in my throat past midnight
                        and your brave tra-la-la
        half a world away
                        it's a lonely thing to do
                        and you couldn't get used to the cold
                                                or the hole in the bed
                        the silence after you sang out
                        the songs that would never mean dancing again

oh my sentimental mother
you died
and I saw you in each other's arms again

an hour from dawn
just as it should have been
my dear

I took your rings and came back to the real
life dance of these years

a song by songs and it seems I don't know all the wor
because you never did

but
here we are driving the coasts of our dreams and
bending again in time

over the precious cradle of the heart

Elizabeth Nannestad

On Love

Let me tell you, it's
all pain.
And there we go, every one of us
time and again.

Take one who's been bitten
badly, left alone.
Chances are
such a one could still be interested
in kissing someone.

It's a slippery slope
neat and sudden.
Your friends shout '*Look out!*' You're
head over heels
and bound to be
smashed at the bottom.

Love is definitely
not kind,
cares nothing
for the mess behind.

Not love, no.
It just carries on
whistling.

Elizabeth Smither

The Lions

The old lion at the zoo
Services the lioness in his cage;
She lies like a stone lion
In every botanic garden
Her eyes grown hazy, hardly moves—
She finds him impetuous and foolish perhaps?
The two great heads, heavy paws
And velvet strung on bone between
Have a classic heavy grace still
In this ridiculous place, next to the
Polar bears always in water like boy scouts.
He leaves a heavy paw on her rump after
Like an evening purse against a golden gown.

Temptations of St Antony by His Housekeeper

Once or twice he eyed me oddly. Once
He said Thank God you're a normal woman
As though he meant a wardrobe and went off
Humming to tell his beads. He keeps
A notebook, full of squiggles I thought, some
Symbolism for something, I think I've seen
It on lavatory walls, objects like chickens' necks

Wrung but not dead, the squawking
Still in the design, the murderer running.
He's harmless, God knows. I could tell him
If he asked, he terrifies himself.
I think it makes him pray better, or at least
He spends longer and longer on his knees.

M.K. Joseph

The Girl Who Stayed at Home

My love put on his battledress
    And then he went away
I kissed him at the station
    But that was yesterday
That was yesterday my love
    And now the tears are dried
And I sit upon the beach
    With a new love by my side.

My love was dressed in navy blue
    The sweethearts in a row
Stood waving from the quayside
    But that was a month ago
Thirty days ago my love
    The heart must keep warm
So I walk in the city
    With a new love on my arm.

My love wore his shining wings
    A speck in the air
I watched him I watched him
    But that was last year
Spring comes again my love
    And now you are dead
And the old pain returning
    And a new love in my bed.

Keith Sinclair

A Night Full of Nothing

We met in a bushel of paradise birds
While the cockatoo langled his whimsical lay.
I garbled her mouth for a wonder of words,
O why did she linger and why did she stay?

Her breasts were a gallon of gathering bees
And lily legs walked her down lover's delay
As we ripened like raspberries high in the trees,
O why did she linger and why did she stay?

She was the mare all a-meadowed with spring
And I was a night-time of lances to slay
In the lists of her limbs, in her laughter my ring
O why did she linger and why did she stay?

We larked it, we liked it, all play-timing on,
It was dripping with moonshine from kiss to doomsday.
One night full of nothing and then she was gone,
O why did she linger and why did she stay?

Ian Wedde

Sonnet for Carlos

After 'Sir Walter Rawleigh to his Sonne'

There are three things Carlos that break into
our world & flourish while they are apart
but sometimes they join forces in the heart
& this dull axis brings us wrack & rue.
The three are these: love, the one, the many.
Love, love it is that lends the beacon light,

our feet grip earth because of solitude,
the many has the power to make us fly.
Ah Carlos, while this tension lasts you'll see
how love burns, earth breathes, sails of heaven soar.
But when that pitch is slack then love will flee.
the earth be clay, & Carlos fly no more.

> *Then bless thee, & beware, & lett us praye,*
> *Wee part not with thee at this meeting daye.*

Elizabeth Spencer

Wife in Wartime

Gone from me, you father of my son,
as feckless peasant casting seed
considers that the work is done.
Foolish man gone off to kill
a cradle crop.
Heed you not the heart
that booms the bell
of breast
and warns it is
the clappered son
it makes
its guest?

I think of you
then bend to kiss
usurping king.

Snuggle-headed
little thing,
it is for me
his small loins burn.
Hunger for hunger
I return.

Jocasta knew a bliss
ambiguous as this.

Keith Sinclair

Fathers and Sons Night

They show two films
on bodily growth
and human procreation.
Greek statues and diagrams
illustrate the track
of hunting sperm
ascending Fallopian tubes,
but not the blind penis,
spear thrust through the wall
of a thatched hut,
bird beak reaming a lily.
The doctor talks fatherly;
he answers questions on v.d.,
describes how twins occur.
Is no-one going to mention
love's blindingness?
flint arrowheads striking home?
and the hurt, the open,
the helpless heart?

Fleur Adcock

The Lover

Always he would inhabit an alien landscape,
Someone else's setting; he walked with surly
Devotion the moist paths of a bush valley
Whose trees had spoken to one he could not keep
As friend; he would learn local names, claim kinship
By an act of will; then let his mind haunt
And cling as hands grasped branches, stones,
Eyes learnt by heart another sky's shape.

In late childhood he had lived a year
Emotionally wedded to an elm, whose leaves
Crumbling in all his pockets evoked rough
And bitter the warm bark; then a small creek

Had filled one summer with the breathing air
Of willows and brown water; by such loving
He cast off abounding more exacting dreams
And baffled others less than he would think.

Later, his enlarging world demanded
Mountains, passionate rivers, a harsh bay,
As wider symbols; where no loved face
Spread to his hand, he would stroke wind-grained wood,
Learn and cherish a stone's contours, and,
Where once the grace of a girl's voice had spoken,
Set blind feet on the hare's path to walk
And closet with a rock his loving blood.

The climax never came; he might have cooled
His flesh utterly in the sudden river,
Or found long satisfaction in a haven
Made solitary by hills; but gradually
The challenging lust ebbed back unfulfilled.
Now, set apart, he lets the city's plan
Absorb him calmly; only now and then
Stares at the harbour, at the vivid sea.

Kate Camp

In Your Absence

In your absence
I stubbed out my arm.

Parcelled myself off
to various chaps.

I put the dog's head in a bucket
and she barked my shin

I put my head down, received
brief papery epiphanies.

Enjoying a thermos of tea
in the Australian Garden

I thought—this is very fine, and—
no one is coming to rescue me.

Anne French

from *New Zealanders at Home*

1 *Autumn*

The sex life of the sheep is at best
perfunctory. Conducted in public,

it is somewhat less a matter of taste
than need, of urgency than absent-

mindedness, of finesse than dull
thrusting. What the ewe thinks

can be guessed from her composure.
She chews steadily throughout

the whole performance, a glazed
look in her yellow eyes. Afterwards

she shambles off to crop the short
autumn grass as though he's kept

her from something. Does he murmur
Was that good for you too? into

her ear when he's done? *Did the earth
move?* His majestic balls swing

as he walks, like spuds in a wet
sack. He might call her later.

James Brown

Map Reference

after Laurie Anderson

I was out walking, when this car
pulled over, and the electric window
wound down. 'Excuse me,'
said the woman inside,
'but I'm new here—

I'm newer than that building over there
and it hasn't even been built.
Yet somehow already I'm lost,
I'm lost in this
big city. Everything I've seen
looks like everything I've seen.
I was looking for Tuesday
I was following the signs
but somewhere must have taken
a wrong turn.
I just kept driving
it all looked sort of familiar.'
Then she smiled.
And her smile was like the swing
of uninterrupted coast line
from forty thousand feet.
I was sure I had seen her
somewhere before.
And I said, 'Perhaps?
Perhaps we could have coffee?'
And she said, 'If only,
if only I had a map, I could find
the centre—or one of them—
and I could just work out.'
She said, 'If only
I could find the right point.'
So I told her I was unemployed,
how I used to know about Tuesday
but that now I only knew about
Saturday and Sunday
—which are sister suburbs
just out of town
where the working tend to go
at weekends.
And she said she may have been there
but just passed straight through
without really knowing—did one of them
have a coffee factory? she asked
without really wanting to know.
Because she used to be married
she said, to a coffee magnate.
They used to drill for coffee
beneath the ground
beneath the forests
beneath the cities.

It was hard work, following the seams
through all that oil.
And her face lit up like the woman
in the cigarette ad.
And the diamonds on her fingers
were like the New York skyline
just at dusk.
'Of course they're only imitation,' she said.
It was like we were glittering in a rock pool
and the cars were waves
washing over us.
'After the seventh wave,'
she said, 'there will be a break
in the flow.' She said, 'Are you with me?'
But I couldn't go. I had lost
something—it had fallen from my pocket.
I had been looking for it all day.
I needed to find it, to remember
or to forget, or to remember to forget.
She said, 'You will accept my card,
before the window winds up
and I depart?'
Then everything happened
just the way she said it would.
First, there was a break
in the flow; then, I was accepting
her card; before the window
wound up and she
departed.
And somehow, it was amazing.
First she said what would happen
and then, it actually happened.
Like a prophecy
being fulfilled.

Robin Hyde

from *Journey from New Zealand*

Young crude country, hard as unbroken shell . . .
She was hard to love, and took strength, like a virgin.
Sometimes, in money or dust, the little farms ebbed away,
Dripping between disconsolate fingers like blood

Of that harsh girl, who would never love you.
But in the cities (old days!)
We could live better, warm and safe as the sparrows
Twittering through the evenings like young sparrows.
Ours was a city, like any city,
But with more, perhaps, of sea and cloud, not long loved.
November tar, ripening, blackened our sandals.
Our city had doorways, too many shut.
Morning and evening, facing the rampant crimson brutes of the light,
Nobody had the beautiful strength to decree:
'Leave your doors open, morning and evening—
Leave your gates wide to the stranger.'
So ours was a city, like any city, but fair.
At seven (still light), the children snuggled down
Like rabbits. The rest sat on in the lamplight,
Sat still or spoke words by their failures.

There is nothing else to tell, but the catkin grass
Strung on pale wires, close to the sea.
Our great rocks fluked like whales;
We loved the dead coal-hulks, did not despise them.
Money was nothing, balloons were much,
The grey mists quiet-breasted as doves.
I knew a green place where the light looked more like trees,
Trees more like diffused and stilly light.
(Green, green be upon your eyes; red in my heart,
The world's troubled colour: for I must awaken.)
Once in the rose parterres my mother stood still and said:
'Man, woman and child; man, woman and child.'
She was born with a restive heart, but grew old.

Ah, too many sparrows twittering into the dawn . . .
The deep, blue and unborn colour.
The dawn should be men's, not your little voices.
It was always too soon to awake, I remember now,
But the world, this and that world,
And the Templar stars in their order said: 'Rise and go.'

Gordon Challis

Poem for Magda

When I am fit to speak of love the words will come
as easily as wheat puts forth its ample grain
or sunlight skips bright stones across a river.

My tongue thus far is husked and makes harsh sound
and shall not sing until I hear the growth of grain,
until I hear your name in all things blessed forever.

When I am fit to speak of love you may be past
your crest of youthful movement and your grace of line.
It will be late to praise you, late to flatter
myself by implication, finder of your eyes.
And there will be no need to find new ways
to ask or tell each other what's the matter.

Charles Brasch

from *In Your Presence*

A Song Cycle

I practise to believe,
And work towards love.
How should I see
Until I study with your eye?

Nothing I know
Unless you answer for me now.
What was I made for
Except to write your signature?

*

My life and death are yours,
Disposer,
My words and my silence;
Yours the ecstasy, yours the anguish of
This life, this death.

*

Far and far away,
Scent of a rose in the wind,
Your voice comes over the wires,

Smoke of mountain fires—
But you and no other, you,
Clear in the drift of day.

And oh, the heart's play,
Exulting of waters loosed,
As word with word conspires.

*

In love, what do we love
But to give and to receive
That love by which we live.

You, loved and known and unknown,
Are the one and only one
World I am chosen to dwell in.

I turn in your day and your night
Pivoting on one thought,
What we are and are not,

That love as evergreen mover
Is our always and our never,
Creator, destroyer, preserver.

James Bertram

To Charles Brasch at Sixty

Once to you, in an ink-stained room in that southern
School we shared, between our books and the world,
'Suddenly out of a faded picture the past
        Broke with its terrible asking.'

I remember the room, perhaps the picture:
And, carved by fire-light, your trecento profile—
Monkish, brooding, the sallow face with the quirky
        Eyebrows, under a convict haircut.

Other moments. That Sunday evening roll-call,
When the Rector, rosy-flushed from Olympus
(Or Waianakarua), cast his quips, and your purer
        Accent visibly piqued the prefects—

Was it a portent? So for me was the sports day
When, in the half-mile, run to a classic finish,
You like Soames kept your smooth stride, scorning
        To gape or roll for a vulgar medal.

A voice, a stance, a style, a vocation—
They were already yours in that time of choosing,
When the future lay open before us,
        And only the past had questions.

Now the years have filled with their usual freightage
Of war and peace, and little enough we looked for—
'Infinite mess and jumble and dislocation'
        We inherit, like Clough and Arnold.

And if now, grown plainer, sadder, more wary,
We may not look for the Just City descending
From heaven on steppe or paddy or tussock,
        Or the heart of man, *nyedotyopa*—

Still, dear Charles, we can claim each other
By that right of a first election:
Hold to the bond that is longest-lasting,
        A kinship of mind and feeling.

And to you, who built your friends into beacons
Along the way, while your path hugged the shade;
You who kept vows of poverty, claiming only
        'A handful of verse, uncertain in shape and style'—

Can I tell you at last on your sixtieth birthday
Just how wrong you were? For we need not flatter
Our oldest friends: they know far too much about us,
        And we know enough about them.

Who, in a time of the making and breaking of poets,
Brought the gift that was his to its true fulfilment?
Who, when shining talents were buried or squandered,
        Husbanded his, like you?

For you were the shy one, the quietest voice among voices
Heard in these islands, when poetry first rang clear
Finding a music, and finding a meaning, divining
        Speech and sight for the tribe.

But how firmly, through that first confident chorus,
How discreetly, you wove your part in the music:
Never straining the note or wrenching the accent,
        Keeping the pitch and time

Of an ear attuned to all the voices of earth;
To a wind out of space, cool on your cheek as on Rilke's:
Tempering always minor profits and losses
        By longer perspectives of art.

B.E. Baughan

from *The Paddock*

from *Song of the White Clover*

We were young—too young, I said,
When he first proposed the plan;
Mother blind, my hands were full;
We could wait awhile to wed?
Andrew smiled, and shook his head,
Took the section, and began,
Working on the road the while,
As he could, to fall and burn.
—Eh! we had a lot to learn.
We were young and hopeful-hearted.
Ten years we've been married now—
But it's twenty since we started.

First, there came his accident:
Weeks of Hospital: next year,
Debt, instead of Bush, to clear!
Then, wet seasons, and he had
No help, and the 'burns' were bad.
Next, his father died, and Don'
Was but quite a laddie, so
Andrew took their farming on,
And his own had just to go.
Then, at length, when years had seen
Mostly all the young ones wed:
When the land was coming clean,
Fences up, and shearing-shed,
Apple-trees in bearing round
Such a well-stock'd garden-ground,

And the homestead all but done,
And the battle all but won:—
Came the big Bush-fire! So then
All was to begin again.

Well, again it *was* begun.
What yon paddocks lack'd in luck
Was made up to you in pluck,
Oh, it was! and patient skill,
Yes, and splendid, stubborn will.

'Twasn't long from that, when first
Mother, and then Father, died.
All the rest were off and settled.
Janet, just, was left beside.
Then: 'I'm warning you; think well!'
Andrew said, 'I'm still behind,
But—O lassie! should you mind?
Could you manage? 'Twill be tough . . .
Could you live in half a home?'
'Yes!' I told him—if 'twas his,
'Half of half would be enough';
And he answer'd, 'Thank God! Come!'

Aunt took Janet for a while,
And I came,—came here! The track
Lost itself in rocks and bogs,
And through grass less green than black
With the pell-mell stumps and logs.
Suddenly it stopp'd—I saw,
Thro' the whips of driving rain,
And a blasted *Rimu*'s boughs,
—Oh! so naked, rough and raw,
Stumps and logs behind, before,
Paddock to the very door—
Just a clearing, and a house.
Some potatoes round it grew,
Here and there, a sapling tree
Was just big enough to see,
That was all, and that was—You!

Inside, Oh! 'twas worse. I mind,
Shelves and doors were all to find,
Only two rooms even lined,
And the stove dump'd down outside.
I was tired—I could have cried!
Andrew stood and look'd at it,
Then he turn'd, and look'd at me
Struggling that he shouldn't see.
'Ay!' says he, 'So little done!'
Oh, that dear, good, grieving face,
And that disappointed tone,
Fire and wine they were within me!—
'No!' I cried, 'So much *begun*!
Why it's just a new-made world
Given to us two to run—
Us, lad! Won't that mend the moan?
Us! not you, nor me alone.'

Did it matter? Not one bit,
When I look'd that way at it.
Ay, thank God! It *was* 'us two!'
After those long years apart,
When we toil'd, and moil'd, and waited,
Solitary, separated,

There we were at last,—at home,
Hand-in-hand, and heart-to-heart,
Sharing, caring, two together—
Nothing that we couldn't weather!

So, we went to work, we two.
Built and blasted, stump'd and sow'd,
Logg'd-up, dug, and drain'd and hoed,
Milk'd, of course, and made the cheese,
Fenced the paddocks, and the road,
Plough'd a bit, and planted trees,
Rear'd the poultry, started bees.
Up at earliest blink of light,
Often with the stars still bright,
He'd be off, to sledge-in wood;
Mostly I'd to bake at night;
And we'd many pricks and pinches—
Progress only came by inches;
But, it came! We said it should!
Yes, we got on, bit by bit,
Fighting every inch of it;
Day by day, and year by year
Saw some blemish disappear,
Something else come clean and clear;
And the kindly creatures kept
At their growing while we slept.
Ay, we'd only fix'd the yards,
Just the week the boy was born
(I remember, as I lay,
Picturing how *he'd* help, some day!);
Two years back, when Jeanie came,
Why, we'd near five hundred shorn!
. . . That first season, when we found
Things were really coming round—
What a hand it seem'd to lend! . . .
Good times follow'd, wool and stock
Up, and steady as a rock—

Till we settled I could send
For poor Janet; yes, and still,
Step by step, we've gone up-hill,
Slow, but sure and steady; till
Andrew rode to Town, to pay
The last shilling, yesterday!

In the evening, coming back,
There I met him, on the track
That we took, those ten years since,
And we rode, this time, all round
That once rough-and-tumble ground.
No need, now, to sigh, or wince,
Choke the tears, or mend a moan—
There lay our Bush Section: grown,
Paddocks, *You!* and all our own.

K.O. Arvidson

There was a Day

There was a day. There was a day
I gave her daffodils. That
was an August day, and I who gave
took beauty. She is older now,
but her age for me is still of that fine spring.
I do her injustices with daffodils
to keep it that way. Light of the blooms,
                          susurrus of their almost
paper trumpets,
                          wince of fingers folding
the florist's waxed bedeckings;
                    memory,
                    fugue,
                    effigy;
memory only,
fugue in manuscript only,
effigy only,
                    these she knows;

the memory of what was possible weighted down,
crushed corms of conversation, the prothalamium
scored on a priceless vellum silent. Silence.
Daffodils. White limbs in the moon. Pavan.
I do her injustices.
There was an August day.
She is older now.

Fleur Adcock

Ancestor to Devotee

What are you loving me with? I'm dead.
What gland of tenderness throbs in you,
yearning back through the silt of ages
to a face and a voice you never knew?

When you find my name in a document
or my signature on a will,
what is it that makes you hold your breath—
what reverent, half-perverted thrill?

'Flesh of my flesh', we could call each other;
but not uniquely: I've hundreds more
in my posterity, and for you
unreckoned thousands have gone before.

What's left of me, if you gathered it up,
is a faggot of bones, some ink-scrawled paper,
flown-away cells of skin and hair . . .
you could set the lot on fire with a taper.

You breathe your scorching filial love
on a web of related facts and a name.
But I'm combustible now. Watch out:
you'll burn me up with that blow-torch flame.

Peter Bland

Settling Down

A parent at twenty! Such desperation:
a family fathered from a schoolboy's
sexual initiation. The trouble was
I couldn't grow grey hairs. From
juvenile delinquency to middle age
in one stray night was too much to take.
I've had to compromise with the State
and learn to grow up less than gracefully.
At thirty I'm thinking of settling down;
a man needs a loan of his own, a roof
over his wig. It's a sound investment.
Anyway, the kids are howling for a house to break
and, frankly, I'm worried about my second childhood.

Alistair Te Ariki Campbell

Lament

O love, the heart of the faithless world
is still. The element she adored has let her
down, and never again will the trumpeting surf
fly her laughter to the shore . . . The shadow
    of her voice lies buried

in the sand, the hands like folded wings lie
limp and heavy, one upon the other,
and the small dark head, too frail to contain
the vast impetuous spirit, lies desolate
    as unpeopled mirrors.

The moon is down—is this her face I hold
in my hands? Let the reeling sky forever
imitate the heart's constriction, let the cold come,
and the sun not at all. But let no harsher sound
    be heard than what the small

waves make with sighing, or the wind
when like a bee at noonday it might slip
into a flower and be folded up . . .
There was something of the moon about her,
        something of alabaster

that on dark shores the sea threw up
warm and breathing for the tide to talk to,
and wherever she went, like an image loved
by a mirror and kept in its brilliant heart,
        a shadow clung to the sands

like this to sun itself and dream all day . . .
O World, O World, where is the pride now,
the warmth, the wildness? Where now the heart
that once was more than sea to all my drownings?
        She was one of Heaven's

Bright Ones. With her I was everywhere aware
of Heaven, everywhere green and glittering
as the tides at the lips of drowning men,
and terrible as her gay and exquisite smile,
        who now lies drowned.

Charles Doyle

My Love Lies Down Tonight

(For Doran)

My love lies down tonight in an unknown country,
long limbs on a lonely bed. I, who would solve
all mysteries in her, all life, but may not
share even the bitten lip or stir in darkness,
send her my loves, limb-love and deep heart's love,
in that dark country where she lies tonight.

What could I wish for, but to watch her move
in a darkened room in white moonlight,
naked and ready to join in our naked world,
our thin-skinned world of ephemeral, tenuous joy;
to leave as our bodies can all lamentation
for the momentary amnesia of loving.

In the long shells of the empty nights I see her,
a shimmer of water in the deserts of my dreams,
something beyond all hope, beyond all grieving.
I would have us shrive each other of all our crimes,
two thieves forgiven by the Christ of our love;
wish that our long moment of lying there

could be to us forever, that she could love me
in that brief moment more than all the world
of dancers and merrymakers precise and charmed
with dazzle of daylight, in single darkness curled.
Take away, my eyes, if you can, the light of morning;
let us lie together in night without end.

Murray Edmond

Go to Woe

I'm glad I found you.
I thought we should talk.
I believed you would understand.
I didn't know what I was letting myself in for.
Not that it wasn't fun. Are you kidding!
Not that some things couldn't have been different.
The bed was too narrow.
The house was too quiet.
The time was too short.
I admire your honesty.
I think it's impossible.
I meant it as a friendly gesture.
I don't know. Sometimes. Why. You have that look.
In your eye.
Even if I knew now what I didn't know then I still don't know if I'd—
I never felt you were hiding anything.
Did you take a bath afterwards?
This was what I saw when I asked myself what the future would be.
Now I'm here.
I'm touched.

Touched?
Touched . . .
It's the way it goes on, went on . . .
Did you plan it, I mean, when you rang did you?
You were excited, you wanted.
I was scared, I wanted.
The soap. The soap felt. I touched. The soap. the soap.
And the soap felt.
The soap smelt.
The soap melt.
I want to know why why keep it up for so long.
Why is one experience so different from another.
Why is something like this important.
You can't be specific.
Grave and specific.
I think you are very warm. Warm and soft. Warm and soft and sensitive.
I feel you are hiding a lot.
For instance, physically, weren't you tired?
You felt better and better as the summer wore on.
You wore less and less.
And grew more and more desperate.
So you said nothing.
Nothing.
What did you do when you came to part?
What did you say? What did you dance?
I can't say. You can't say.
Free.
Free.
Didn't you say free?
No. Not me.
I thought.
By free you mean alone.
Alone.
Alone and in love.
In love and walking.
Walking and stopping to look in the shop windows.
Watching yourself.
The books, the brandy, the clouds moving past the curtain.
The night moon catching their silver bellies.
There was no moon.

Ruth Dallas

Tinker, Tailor

Tinker, tailor, who can show,
Who that passes can discover
Of old men seated in a row
Which was the deserted lover,
Soldier, sailor, who can tell
Hero now from ne'er-do-well?

Sooner that young mother find
Who can in sun or firelight see
A man grown old and deaf or blind
In the child upon her knee.

Silk, satin, who can trace
In a slow and heavy tread,
See in some old woman's face
The girl who danced the moon to bed,
Is there no one that can tell
Now the wallflower from the belle?

Find two lovers deep in grass
Who can see themselves grown old,
Summer into autumn pass,
And their love turn winter cold.

A Girl's Song

When love came
              glancing
                      down our street
Scarlet leaves
          flew
              round our feet,

    sang the girl, sewing.

He told me
        he would
                come again

Before
        the avenue
                turned green,

  sang the girl, sewing.

How could I know,
                    or guess,
                            till now

The sadness
        of a
            summer bough,

  sang the girl, sewing.

Vivienne Plumb

Journey to the Centre

Speak to me in a language
I cannot understand, I do not want
to understand anything:
akhir cerita itu sedih
the end of the story is sad.

Full of fear one day, cocky the next,
the wind sighs and yawns,
a spider as big as a fifty cent piece
scuttles across the creamy carpet,
trouble comes in threes.
In the bank my spanking new single account
is delivered and entered into the system.

The agapanthus buds are beautiful
penis tips, I think about what
he'll be doing to her now, her lush flesh
like the advertisement *we are all tomatoes*
and must hydrate our skin.
I am the owner of only rotten pieces
of that red fruit, and ignored
in the bottom of my fridge bin
they collapse and subside into their own skins.

But I want to be like those unemployed bums
on the back seat of the bus, drinking and
smelling and singing at ten in the morning.
Love: Oh, I wish for some of that and I spoon
thick brown manuka honey down my sore throat.

When I was three I cried at the Odeon
watching *Journey to the Center of the Earth*,
a quick trip to the inner core,
that journey can be so dangerous.
Where is my medical bandaid?
I am still looking for my fix-it kit
while the credits fade.

Lauris Edmond

Late Starling

Yes yes of course I am hard to please—
yet I can see this quiet sky
with the evening in it
and that poised drop of darkness
the late starling
that comes to the dead peak
of the old pine. Yes, and taste too
the tart smoke of the leaves,
ghost of the year's green,
observe Tortle the cat
slow-stepping across
the darkening grass,
and the single golden pear,
huge and alone, that hangs like a yellow
lantern on its bare branch.

Once we would have stood, my hand in yours,
quiet too, and full of wonder—
was it spring, perhaps, those other evenings?
I have forgotten.
I only know that we have come
to quarrelling, and not even this
communicable peace
can speak to us now.

Tony Beyer

The Ornamentalists

love is an interesting city
to visit in the company
of someone you will
soon be best friends with

white suits and shoes are
of course obligatory
and a red banded panama
you wear in your hand

or set before you on the
café table to watch
the local sun as fat as mercury
that bowls around its crown

there is a beach of boys
of the sort your mothers
warned you both
about turning out like

and the ruins in the moonlight
promise exactly that
if you go alone and late
with your shirt undone

Anne French

Collisions

'Of course she's still intransigent,' you said
between bites as though it isn't someone's marriage.
So I took a good thirty seconds to digest it.
'Intransigent nothing.' Sounds as though I was
their counsellor from Marriage Guidance and not
—well, something similar, if less honourable. More
involved. His consolation, her confidante.
A reflex triangle, you might call it, kinked
briefly backwards against gravity.

How much of that you know I daren't assess,
but note the stillness of your eyes, your voice
as we defend them to each other. It's the boys'
team against the girls'. Result: a draw.
We call it off with a point each on the board.

So do you know it all then, or just what he
told you—not quite the same thing—the plot
and some of the dialogue, with a critical commentary
throughout? Not, presumably, how it happened:
the usual collisions of people from a small
country living in a provincial town.
The predictable, in other words, just waiting
for its chance. I was the meat, that's all—he'll
have told you gristle. Or how it ended: dinners
together, celebrations, people left on planes,
assorted fictions stayed intact. Now silence.
It's relief. But forget his elegant phrases, grand
evoked emotion. Let me risk the awkward
truth—it seems (improbably) I loved them both.

Sam Hunt

A Long Time

A long time now and everyone
lets us know what they think best,
tells us what we should have done—
stay together, love; or bust.

We're given a final warning
today after a long time talking;
and in the mist of the morning
my love and I go walking.

Hone Tuwhare

Humming

(for Kereihi)

It is a house to be constructed with care
    for it has no confining walls
    thus permitting expansion: vertical

    growth is not inhibited for there
    is no limit to the height of the ceiling
    stretching to heaven. This house
    can endure given a chance, that's
    for sure . . . H m m m m

But since it is of earth its foundations may be
    built of sand: and because there are
    no confining walls this fragile house
    of love may be seen as layers of light
    and colour—a feeling tone—warm, purple
    orange grey hot and cold with lots of blue
    and yellow to make it green—green
    and predictable . . . H m m m m

Fleshed out though, this house of love isn't
    ageless, but aged old. It has form; contour.
    It has presence; a brilliant arc uniting
    heaven and hell; love-thoughts in pursuit of
    a physical expression—a noisy, gloppy
    proclamation—

        Aha   Aha—Aha—Aha   Aha

    . . . and horses, huffing and pounding into
    the straight, riders snarling, cruel whips
    flailing—the anguish of stretched leather
    reeking sweetly of sweat . . . And reason? Ahhh.

    Reason is a hunchback of irrelevance backing
    quietly out the door.

But where are the flowers—the select flowers
    of endearment, soul-food to dazzle the heart?

    O, they're here, all right: there, there
    and THERE . . . H m m m m

Vincent O'Sullivan

Elegy, of Sorts

I come into a room with its deep leather chair
and I say, 'Death, can't you stand for a bit,
let a man who is tired take his turn sitting down?'

Darkness the size more or less of the average human
lumbers aside. Manners don't come into it, mind you.
It's of no great concern. Time is on his side.

Then he says from behind me—no one, need
I say, has seen his mouth move—he says
'It is so easy to love hair like this, isn't that so,

when a woman's young and alive?' and he shakes
the brilliant skein over his forearm the way you see
carpet vendors stroke what they have to offer,

as if letting it go's the last thing they could bear.
And I forget he is even there, his immeasurable patience . . .
I think of each minute as a single thread, a single

strand, then the crop is swept up by a broad advancing
hand, and the treasure is someone else's, or no one's,
or God's. But by then the name you used

is downstream, its dye in the current, is of no
relevance to the world of lines, of snares, of restraining nets . . .
There is a song that used to go, 'Your eyes,

my sister, crack open my heart.' And a dance
that went with it, spread from stone to stone,
and at the end, after the music, after the train

of silence that follows music, you knew was a song
about a woman's hair, although her name is one
of a million words the song does not include.

Lauris Edmond

The Names

Six o'clock, the morning still and
the moon up, cool profile of the night;
time small and flat as an envelope—
see, you slip out easily: do I know you?
Your names have still their old power,
they sing softly like voices across water.

Virginia Frances Martin Rachel Stephanie
Katherine—the sounds blend and chant
in some closed chamber of the ear, poised
in the early air before echoes formed.
Suddenly a door flies open, the music
breaks into a roar, it is everywhere;

now it's laughter and screaming, the crack
of a branch in the plum tree, the gasping
and blood on the ground; it is sea-surge
and summer, 'Watch me!' sucked under
the breakers; the hum of the lupins, through
sleepy popping of pods the saying of names.

And all the time the wind that creaked in
the black macrocarpas and whined in the wires
was waiting to sweep us away; my children who
were my blood and breathing I do not know you:
we are friends, we write often, there are
occasions, news from abroad. One of you is dead.

I do not listen fearfully for you in the night,
exasperating you with my concern,
I scarcely call this old habit love—
yet you have come to me this white morning,
and remind me that to name a child is brave,
or foolhardy; even now it shakes me.

The small opaque moon, wafer of light,
grows fainter and disappears; but
the names will never leave me, I hear
them calling like boatmen far over
the harbour at first light. They will sound
in the dreams of your children's children.

Part 5

Our long voyaging

A.R.D. Fairburn

Poem

Age will unfasten us, and take our strength;
our world will end when you,
the lovely husk of love, lie still at length
on the cold bed, and I,
my limbs stained through and through
with your beauty's blood, powerless beside you lie.

The world was old when we awoke
in this rebirth, and looked our love, and spoke;
the moon, white seal upon our midnight bliss,
a desert ages old at our first kiss.
Time will devour our days,
love die before we die.
Dear girl, when the dawn no longer finds us close
and sleeping still, wrapped in one dream,
Heaven's air around; when we,
rising in sunlight, gaze
no more on the enriched earth, but see
dust on the leaves and thin
light from the famished sun, and feel
the dryness of the heart;
then will our world be past, and a new age begun,
wherein we sleep and have no part.

And I would come up singing from the south,
or rise through smothering tides of sleep
deep as the sea, and find your mouth,
and lie there motionless till we became
(O flame and shadow of remembered time!)
one shape, one thought, the living form
of love itself; then slip beneath the wave
still warm from you, still crying your name.

A Farewell

What is there left to be said?
There is nothing we can say,
nothing at all to be done
to undo the time of day;
no words to make the sun
roll east, or raise the dead.

I loved you as I love life:
the hand I stretched out to you
returning like Noah's dove
brought a new earth to view,
till I was quick with love;
but Time sharpens his knife,

Time smiles and whets his knife,
and something has got to come out
quickly, and be buried deep,
not spoken or thought about
or remembered even in sleep.
You must live, get on with your life.

William Hart-Smith

Smoke Signal

No, you can never be lost to me
even if I do not know
exactly where you are
but it's better if my eyes go
searching in one direction

hand over brow
like a blackfellow

for I do like to know
approximately
where you are
and what you may be doing
so that I may look and see

far away to the south
a thin blue thread
of smoke rising
so inconspicuous and still
it could have gone unnoticed

then I can concentrate
and think the thoughts you think
and smell the fragrance of your skin
and taste the taste of your mouth.

William Hart-Smith

Postage Stamp

If you should ever have to
part from someone dear, tear
yourself away, be sure

the tear is where
the perforations are. Please,
please do not ever

recklessly sever, sheer
yourself from some one other
so that their stamp is torn

and you have part of their
living, bleeding
flesh at your side worn.

Michael Morrissey

Movie Madonnas

Wounds of Christ
Are not more saintly than the delicate
Tracery of crimson from your lips

I salute you Heroines of B grade grief!
Your handkerchiefs are wet with intelligence
You know far more than we

When the blood and rosed affair of Romanticism
Ceases to 'drive light up your spines'
You will come to our 'emotional rescue'

Your wash of tears permit our guilt

Pat Wilson

The Farewell

And so, one day when the tide was away out,
The gulls there dancing along the edge of the sea,
We walked across the sand, down to the boat
And began again—she to protest and appeal,
I to refuse, looking aside, and then turning
And smiling . . .

        for it was not as if I had
Whatever it was that she asked, but who could persuade her
Of that? nor was it true that I could pretend
For ever . . .

       and all the gulls there, crying and playing,
Hunting, and all the reds and browns and yellows
Of late afternoon, and the last tints of the blue
Going out with the tide, and the boat drawn up there fast
Becoming high and dry on the sand as we talked.

Elizabeth Smither

A Cortège of Daughters

A quite ordinary funeral: the corpse
Unknown to the priest. The twenty-third psalm.
The readings by serious businessmen
One who nearly tripped on the unaccustomed pew.
The kneelers and the sitters like sheep and goats.

But by some prior determination a row
Of daughters and daughters-in-law rose
To act as pallbearers instead of men
All of even height and beautiful.
One wore in her hair a black and white striped bow.

And in the midst of their queenliness
One in dark flowered silk, the corpse
Had become a man before they reached the porch
So loved he had his own dark barge
Which their slow-moving steps rowed
As a dark lake is sometimes surrounded by irises.

W.H. Oliver

The Swineherd

They are all love stories. Some are subversive,
notably the one of the prince who pretended
to be a swineherd, and of the covetous girl
with a passion for music, toys and cunning
instruments. He named and exacted his price
and rejected her utterly. But, the consequences!
Later, still bored, he went away on crusade.
The lady followed disguised as a young esquire.
They took the wrong turning for the Holy Land
and came to a stop somewhere in Asia Minor,
guests of a community of heretics
whose pastor, white beard yellow about the mouth,
quickly unstitched all the articles of belief
they had ever entertained, especially those
touching upon the possession of property,
dignities, distinctions, orders of precedence,
decorum and protocol, showing them to be both
untrue and of a mischievous tendency.
The mechanical bird flew off to the oleanders
and refused to sing any more. The prince
wound himself up like a toy and delivered
quite excellent music. She listened entranced
until she could no longer hold it all in her heart
and switched him off in mid-cadence.
Behind his great beard the pastor of the heretics
smiled to himself, a yellow wintry smile,
rehearsing another sermon on the celibate state.
She reckoned he would, in his turn, sing sweetly enough.

Ursula Bethell

from *Six Memorials*

October 1935

The green has come back, the spring green, the new green,
Darling, the young green upon the field willows,
And the gorse on the wild hills was never so yellow,
Together, together, past years we have looked on the scene.

The loved little bird is singing his small song,
Dearest, and whether the trill of the riro
Reminded, we wondered, of joy or of sorrow—
Now I am taught it is tears, it is tears that to spring time belong.

You were laughter, my liking, and frolic, my lost one,
   I must dissemble and smile still for your sake,
   Now that I know how spring time is heart-break,
Now you have left me to look upon all that is lovely, alone.

James K. Baxter

On the Death of Her Body

It is a thought breaking the granite heart
Time has given me, that my one treasure,
Your limbs, those passion vines, that bamboo body

Should age and slacken, rot
Some day in a ghastly clay-topped hole.
They led me to the mountains beyond pleasure

Where each is not gross body or blank soul
But a strong harp the wind of genesis
Makes music in, such resonant music

That I was Adam, loosened by your kiss
From time's hard bond, and you,
My love, in the world's first summer stood

Plucking the flowers of the abyss.

Leonard Lambert

My Early Love

My early love was a child in endless pursuit of cold afternoons.
My love was intermittent patches of black and purple against
deep green trees near dusk; in the liquid night an uncertain
whiteness, with the Moon abroad to sprinkle plausibility on
my dreams, spear with hope my longing.

My love was a school before and after the presence of children.

Her smile sometimes would beat against the near horizons
of my timid life, opening to me vast richly textured worlds,
awakening impossible loves.

Elizabeth Nannestad

La Strada

Let us call it love: your absences, your violence.
Take this in reply, a poem less flattering than the rest
I seal with my sort of love and send
towards a little man on a long road.

The people you meet, in their tents and their towns,
are actors, people whose faces light up
before they turn around, forget you, and go home.
What you go looking for I daresay you will find.

I know what you'll say,—what does she know? She exaggerates.
And so I do. Your everlasting meanness rules our lives,
your freedom by now worth nothing.
What do you want from me? Remember—I don't lend. I give.

Sunshine on a plain wall. I know it's there.
My skin knows it, and knows when it is gone.
That is what I like: the sun. And when
it is gone, I mind. But not for long.

Eventually God will dispose of us. He will
give us a number. We forget almost everything
and later, too, will forget what it was like to be side by side,
to lie and listen to your fist of a heart opening.

Kate Camp

Dear Sir

I have received your visit and comments, with regret.
I am always disappointed to lose a lover,
especially a long-standing lover like yourself,
and I'd like to take this opportunity to thank you for your past
    contribution.
I enclose a list of our recent sexual encounters,
which I hope will be of interest.

Regarding your concerns about our relationship,
I can certainly sympathise with your position.
However, like most things in life,
relationships are not simple,
and I can assure you
that my policies have been decided
after careful consideration
of the best available science.

This correspondence is now closed.

Anne French

Parallel Universes

(after the book by Fred Alan Wolf)

It's a relief to learn that after all
this is not the only time–space
continuum. That there is another
parallel universe, in which you
love me quite as tenderly as I love
you, in which we are together and happy.
Also one in which you don't, but
are prepared to keep trying. And
another in which I gave up on you
long since, and another in which
we hardly know each other, and
still more in which neither of us

will ever be born, let alone make
each other miserable. We are carried
forward into a radiant array of possible
futures on the quantum wave of
probabilities. At last, spiralling
down into a singularity, I understand
you perfectly and forgive you everything.

Hugh Lauder

Silence

When you left:
silence.
Others followed saying you would not return.

Imagine the water's
curving arc, falling and landing
beyond sound.

This is how it felt
thinking of you
and now you are gone
and will not return.

When I am called
I stand quite still
waiting for the noise
to clear.

The Descent

'*così bello viver di cittadini . . . così dolce ostello*'
Paradiso, *XV: 130, 132*

It is a spring dawn,
it is the wrong century.

                                        Here
                        on the edge of Florence
                        we shall sleep
                        through the summer
                        dream of what
                        we have forgotten.
                        Guns cradled
                        in our locked arms.

                        The stones of history
                        are not so strong
                        we have pounded them
                        into rubble;
                        here a fresco's fragment
                        shows the carnal love
                        between wolf and man,
                        and there, the inscriptions
                        of a dead tongue.

                        We have come far
                        from the memory
                        of flight.
                        Soon we shall
                        sleep,
                        feathers falling
                        like ash.

Patuwhakairi

Lament for Ngaro

The evening star is setting
Over the ridge at 'Ati Rau.
What is left to me now my love is gone?
You were my great treasure!
Girl who is far distant, who fled,
Went so fast in the light of day,
The rays of the sun, you were a rustling cabbage tree
In Awapoka, where you used to roam!
Oh you disappeared, went suddenly—
You did not pause, your heart was set on going!

Put on your garment as the dawn comes up
That your people may set out for
The entrance to the earth, and Maui's precious thing
May be seen above, and be gathered in—
The heaped-up produce of your relatives!
The daughter of Rau must go speedily—
You must dive for mussels sleeping on the rocks
And catch fish that pluck the seaweed, to be thrown down
As food to be strung together by your people—
The company of women, the multitude of Titoro!

Where now are the western tides?
She is gone, my prop of the rising tides,
My prop of the ebbing tides that lie beyond
The beaches by the sea, where her companions stand!
Go out in a canoe that glides in the wind,
Meet the current spread out before you,
Then swim, for it is the wide ocean!
Flocks of godwits are gathering,
Moving restlessly on the seaward cliffs!
You were bound to us, our best beloved!
Oh why was your fallen head so sacred
It was not given to us, who would have greeted it
With tears in this world!

Kendrick Smithyman

Still Life

All the others laugh nastily.
They run away. She is left, pudgy girl
child surrounded by distance.
They know how; she does not know how.
She doesn't want to cry. Bewildered,
where there are many problems,
her hands twist a hair ribbon that's worked loose.
She is unlovely. She can never make up her mind,
what to do with her hands. Love is not
impossible. Love runs away, stealing
all the names in the world, leaving only
distance and hands
which cannot pick up pieces of laughter,
or names.

'What is turbot?' she asks the assistant
at the supermarket's delicatessen.
And, 'Where does turbot come from, smoked?'
If smoked, 'What do you do with it? It's
twenty-nine cents.'

Marry yourself to sickness, call sickness
Wife, Husband, for better or worse
who has no name and was not standing
beside her. Here is a problem. It costs
not quite thirty cents and who would hang
a packaged fish upon a tree
as though that would be any answer, finally?

Her hands don't bother to tell. They are busy
with their own life. Besides, trees are
where leaves dry out thin, like fading
laughing voices. Trees were for
birds which did not carry names in their mouths
like children. Yet when she notices
the sparrow which flew into the market
and perched on a rafter over fruits
you just about smell the fear
coming off her. Love is not
impossible, only unlikely. Some have a flair
for loving, as others are good with names.

Rachel McAlpine

How to Live Without Love

You have to inform the Post Office,
the City Council and the Bank.
They will promptly rush you with geraniums.

Then you look at your children. Yes.

You make a calendar of friends:
it all adds up. Today,
an unexpected fuck, a bonus
you'll regret tomorrow—
count your blessings.

A stranger is on the way
to provide a ludicrous fantasy.
This week you'll get a cuddle
or a nice cup of tea.
Have you noticed I'm holding your hand?

Cicadas work on their physique
for years before they join
the orchestra.
Pohutukawas hang on tight
and know this year they're due
for the big red bloom.
There's one working itself up now;
you can't imagine it lending
more than its equity,
not to Latin America, anyway.

I haven't convinced you yet,
I see
halfway through your adult life
two likely endings: twenty-five years
of blunders under blankets, or
a single suitable face,
alarming with love.

This summer the hills are silent.
Next year courting may be raucous.
Stop trying to die:
it's much too soon, it's lazy.

James Brown

A New Position

Inside the lost elation
of a foreign room, I found
just how easy it was.
To make and break.

Nothing ever really isn't, is it?
Or is—signed, sealed, *and* delivered
properly intact. But then,
I would say that.

It is an unaccustomed position,
not being victim. Oh I 'the baddie'
felt bad, had my sorrow.
But nothing like you.

The truth was cold
and told me how I can't
have *really* liked you so much.
Seems you were right.

Of course, I didn't mean to,
never intended—all of that.
Promises, then and now, collapse
your face.

I cry too
for you, for me and my
terrible new power.
Honest tears.

But in the end I leave.
Decide I will take up my
new position. I mean,
this could be the one.

Katherine Mansfield

The Meeting

We started speaking—
Looked at each other; then turned away—
The tears kept rising to my eyes
But I could not weep
I wanted to take your hand
But my hand trembled.
You kept counting the days
Before we should meet again
But both of us felt in our heart
That we parted for ever and ever.
The ticking of the little clock filled the quiet room—
Listen I said; it is so loud
Like a horse galloping on a lonely road.
As loud as that—a horse galloping past in the night.
You shut me up in your arms—
But the sound of the clock stifled our hearts' beating.

Elizabeth Nannestad

You Must Be Joking

I waited for you until the hours turned to stone
I came as agreed, you left me alone.

Now you have lost the expression
of furious impatience you saved for me:

'I had forgotten you were so gentle'

Oh then I loved you like the sun

But that was then, my friend, and now
By my ambition and my family name

By the brother I lost and the will I own
By the wind there on the street where I stood

You can call, you can call. I will not come.

Kevin Ireland

from Six Songs for Soprano

1 The Professor of Love

the Professor of Love
in the lecture hall
talked of his descent to Hell

he coached the students
for an hour
on: I am the Outrage and the Power

he tossed the textbooks
in the air
and tore his gown and smashed a chair

and warned the throng
who sought instruction
in the arts and skills of self-destruction

that conjugate it
how you will
In Love means: falling
                    fallen
                        fall

Andrew Johnson

In White

She came so close—so curious—
he thought he'd caught the scent of her thinking.

She said her heart, a bird—in white—
had long since left the nest, because it was restless

and hadn't returned
so he built a screen in white

around her heartlessness:
these are the hopeless movies he projected

because she offered nothing
and he accepted.

Keith Sinclair

The Furies

The Furies have immense intelligence:
ask why to every question,
cross-question each nuance—
'Last night you said . . .
but now you say . . .'
Their moral scruples are insatiable:
they tear their men to pieces
before they go to bed.
In bed they fling themselves
and their tormented men
far out upon the wildest sensual swings
and afterwards they hack at them again
with doubts, denials, blame.
They have to analyse, these holy sluts,
each glance and touch.
There is in their hysteric world no time
for kindnesses like kissing afterwards.

Elizabeth Smither

To Write of Love

One day to write of love he set
A brandy glass and a rose
Beside the typewriter and half a ream
Of white paper. It was too perfect
What could he find to say?
He had intended speaking
Of claypits hung over with roses
The climbing sort, himself climbing out
Grasping the briars, stung but lured on
By the ferocious scent. He got to the top
And lay on the wet grass, his hands all
Bleeding. He looked down at his hands
They were cured. He could type 50 words a minute
But none came. So he poured a brandy.

Michael Jackson

A Marriage

In a room of black enamel, gold
filigree, two schemed to love;
often must they have been like us,
one stood at this window looking down
into a maze, the clouded waters of
the moat, the other recollected
something of that first far meeting,
a hunting party in the White Chateau
and the cold hills near Orleans.

Now it is all embellishment, grace
of swans, eglantine under snow
and barking hounds, is woven on
the legendary cloth that hangs
upon the spontaneity of dawn;
by a lucid river, how could our love
go on? I turn from reverie
to welcome you, in whom the sound
of hunting in the forest ends
a pale fox dead on a green lawn.

Fille de Joie: Congo

Lips caked with lipstick
And the smell of booze
You dance with the man of ten thousand francs
Until the music moves him to
Take you to the room where the rite will be.

Preferring him not
To put out the light
You remove a bonnet of dead women's hair
Beneath which you jealously preserve
Stiff twirls of the African coiffure.

Down to your silken underthings
Breasts astir
And his own undoing scarcely seen
You are the cur under midnight heat
Of a mad dog doing it
For what in Europe would have been love.

Louis Johnson

from *Sonnets—More or Less*

3 *Remainders*

We ceased to grow together. You achieved
some point of status that was satisfied
with being where it was, and flaunted that
as trophy for your family and friends.
For us, though, talking ended. Quiet nights
in which you planned new chores and fresh assaults
on the next morning turned to spit and polish,
the busy hiss of frying time. At parties
we'd meet as strangers, sometimes like each other.
I heard you talking once about a man
who seemed of interest. He turned out to be me,
but I did not know him. At home
he took you to bed for a turn of tender loving
and woke wet-faced. By daylight he had gone.

4 Nisi

It is knowing what to leave out. Curt messages,
notes left on the dressing-table count
as a failure of speech. By noon it will need
full legal letters and the assembled court
to decide what is essential shall be heard
and judgement taken. White-wigged ghosts
in the ante-rooms of choice hover and thumb
texts. But we have still not spoken. Pale
eyed, we have become not ourselves but acts
engineered by others out of theory. Images
speak for us: walk out in a dream stricken
with screams from the dungeons. A quill
or a knife make sense by dividing the ring
that bound. Blood flows from a severed finger.

Helen Jacobs

The Ice of Kindness

I do not think we will explore
            each other more
            but rest
on what we have touched together,
having come to kindness
            gently.

And I will fail you over and over
            turning outwards
            my competence,
not asking you to say what
you need me to reveal you
            to say.

So we will both walk softly
            on the ice
            of kindness,
which with care may last
across the dark water out
            our days.

R.A.K. Mason

Our Love was a Grim Citadel

Our love was a grim citadel:
>no tawdry plaything for the minute
>of strong dark stone we built it well
>and based in the ever-living granite:

The urgent columns of the years
>press on, like tall rain up the valley:
>and Chaos bids ten thousand spears
>run to erase our straw-built folly.

Lugete o Veneres

With his penis swollen for the girl on the next farm and rigid
>here he lies on his bed
motionless dumb and his naked corpse goose-fleshed and as frigid
>as if he were dead:

Only at times a great sob rises up in his drawn aching throttle
>and dies like his hope
or the tear of his anguish drips down on his arm cold and mottled
>like a bar of blue soap.

For the people next door have packed up their pots and their table
>and their mats and their ploughs
they have brought up their pigs from the sty their steeds from the stable
>and driven off the cows.

Tomorrow strange people will reign there tomorrow the stranger
>will inherit their places
other cows know the shed where they milk, new horses the manger
>and dogs with unknown faces.

Mark how dejected tormented he lies poor lad while shivers
>run and shake his fat arse;
for a space let us mourn here this tortured boy's slobbering quivers
>as we laugh at the farce.

M.K. Joseph

Cinderella

She was content in the kitchen, hugging cheap dreams
Until that old woman, starting in a puff
Of ashes, clothed her in cobweb and moonbeams,
Conjured a coach from rats and kitchen-stuff.
At midnight the dress upon the dancing-floor
Lay dirt and glimmer, the slippers were ice-hard,
The clock-prince chimed along the corridor,
She fled him weeping through the palace-yard.
But the old witch had her way; the messengers
Went out to match the slipper to the true princess.
Dragged in her rags before the tittering courtiers,
Put to the question, she could only whisper *Yes*.
In glass-heeled slippers she minces towards the tomb
Beside her bridegroom ticking like a bomb.

Koenraad Kuiper

from *Addresses*

II *To His Mistress*

It's thoughtful of you to come and see me;
None of the others have (I suppose he told you).
It's a compliment perhaps or are we getting older
more sensitive of time,
not that it has changed him you understand.
But we do share something else,
you and I, his weaknesses, and you have come
to share it with me
as if I have too much.

I haven't now and never have had you should know.
There was a time when children made it up,
the gaps I mean.

And now here are we talking of him
for want of something else.

Leonard Lambert

Cold Eyes

For Christine

1

We were easy in the aisle of a great crowded theatre.
Judging stares we met with a cold open gaze.
Nobody guessed how very very old we were.
How shocked they would have been to learn
Of our deadly subversions.

2

I followed you everywhere, loving your intricate
Mysterious turnings. We questioned nothing.
Time let us be.
To some I think we appeared as small saviours.
There were cheers in their eyes
As they watched the unfolding of our legend.
From their chains & narrow prisons they waved
Encouragement.
How I loved the way no explanation
Could quite catch you, a flashing tangent
To all established directions.

3

Then somewhere you turned too quickly.
Or maybe I betrayed you. Anyhow there came
A bulk of world between us
And I had somehow thickened & stiffened
And grown somewhat taller.
Did they get you I wonder.
What a time.
Goodbye Cold Eyes.

Wilhelmina Sherriff Elliott

Nga Huia

This was the musing of Pomare's daughter,
Queen-like Nga Huia, in far Whangaroa:

I am thine only, my Pakeha husband,
Only and always, for ever and ever.
Gone from me, beautiful! gone from me, brave one!
Gone with thy warriors to fierce Whanganui!
Leaping wave, swelling sail, joying to bear thee;
Sun, moon, and stars, all rejoicing to serve thee;
Ah! but I, too, must exult in thy presence!
How can I linger bereft of my heart's blood?

So with next dawning arose the young princess,
Met the great chiefs of the noble Nga Puhi,
All but the greatest, her father, held captive
Out on the war-ship: the thunderous *North Star.*

Proudly she listened to stories of rivers
Foaming infuriate over huge boulders;
Stories of forest, untracked, never ending;
Stories of sulphurous horrible mud-holes;
Stories of mountains, which, devil-tormented,
Fling in the face of high heaven their blasphemings,
Pour on earth's fair tender breast maledictions;
Proudly she listened, and answered them only:
All this, and more, will I dare for my hero!

On, gallant horse! with your strong steady paces,
Hundreds of miles stretch untravelled before you:
Maunga Kahia, Wairoa, Kaipara,
Bright Waitemata, and rolling Wakiato,
Taupo Moăna, and then Ahuriri;
Tribe telling tribe of the wonderful journey,
Braved for the first time, so grandly, so fondly:
Sixty young chiefs riding out from Otaki—
Cavalcade royal for pioneer royal—
Honour and gladness around her, within her,
Thus Whanganui was reached by Nga Huia!

Sweet, sweet the heart-song deliciously chanted
All through the glowing emparadised seasons;
Lovely the floweret that burst into being,

Fair as her kindred in old English gardens:
Beautiful *Nota*, in soft-vowelled Maori:
North Star, in baptism and holy thanksgiving.

Letters from Home, from the old English gardens:
Come to inherit a great benefaction!

Ah! the bewailing, the pitiful pleading,
Promises perjured, and eager departure;
Evil days, frantic nights, one ray delusive
Torturing on to the blackness of darkness;
Never the summons came, never the token,
Only an oversea chatter belauding
Elwes, his mansion, and wide cultured acres.

Out from the chasm of her soul's desolation
Huia yearned northward to father and people:
Journeyed again the wild length of the island;
Bearing her innocent sweet golden lily;
Wearing the image, her tribe's richest jewel,
Once, as her love gift, a sign of devotion.
where she gave all in majestic confiding.

Now the heitiki becomes your atua,
Pomare muttered, *and death is its omen!*
Low drooped the stately head, faded the glory
Of each resplendent charm, faded the sorrow:
Nga Huia ceased from Te Ika a Maui!

Soon, weary Pomare, savage but faithful,
Doomed in his love and pride, slain by her anguish,
Laid his great heart in the grave of his daughter!

Auē! thrice-orphaned! auë! Nota Elwes!
Scarce had the century mounted its zenith,
(Lurid and ominous now in its setting!)
When that frail infancy quivered to knowledge,
Woke to mortality's bitterest questions:
Craft and ferocity coldly triumphant,
Strength growing stronger by fierce spoliation,
Piteous need amid opulent birthright,
Mutual hatreds throughout man's dominion.

Problem inscrutable? Nay; the solution
Gleams through the mists of the loneliest sorrow,
Hints of far different stages of being:
Cause that shall win a divine vindication—

Failure that truly is shining achievement—
Time but a beat in eternity's rhythmus—
Love the one verity, one consummation!

Charles Spear

Audrey

You fly a kite against a silver sky;
Your tranquil loveliness, pale by the wane
Of sighing tides, gleams like a butterfly
White-crystal-winged in slanting straws of rain.

Sam Hunt

Bottle to Battle to Death

(for Kristin)

From Bottle to Battle to Death,
the places where we lived from
meeting up one champagne night to
splitting up—a child in tow—
one nightmare of an afternoon.

Bottle Creek was our first home,
a boathouse perched on stilts.
The heron thought us one of them.
We paced the mudflats; full tide, swam:
no place (they said) to bring a baby up in.

To Battle Hill where once, one
hundred years before you or I were born,
a poet of a chief held back the Poms.
He let the land fight for him.
Our child was born here. Tom.

Those days, some days, were good,
the nappies flapping at the clouds,
the clouds crash-landing on the hills.
And white as mushrooms on the slopes,
the sheep; at lambing-time, the hawk.

We gave our child Kahu for
a second name, in honour of that hawk.
Our silences invaded us—
the dark hills, sky, the hovering.
It was, for us, an end of talk.

The move then down the valley,
back beside the estuary, the ancient
homestead, Death (and not D'arth!).
We didn't stand a chance.
We stalked each other, minute by minute.

I watched the shy pukeko. They
would run out on the road, crazy as
the clouds that charged the hills.
The cars would always win the game.
Pukeko dead, a dull blue flame.

And then, of course, there was you.
And to say I loved you was true.
And that I hated you was true.
I thought though, if we lie down,
lie down low, we may come through.

Instead, minute by minute, we stalked
each other out. Sometimes we walked
the hills together, Tom in the back-pack,
the dog forever chasing sticks.
And an afternoon, quite casually, I talked

of 'going our own ways'. I can't
remember now what brought me to it.
Perhaps you said, we can't go on this way.
Or, maybe best we call it all a day.
I don't know now. But you went away.

Robin Hyde

from *The People*

II

How she grew old happened in fine-darned places,
Cracked pictures, seen too close; you'd barely know . . .
She was a red-haired woman, two little lines
Sharp cut between her brows: her eyes looked tired
As long as I remember, and her strong mouth sad.
Still she held firmly: when we went for walks
It was I who flagged: You'd never guess what frocks
She made us, while the clean thread broke and broke,
And I stood pricking at red sateen, or spoke
Roughly: that dance, the only one we had,
I remember Judy's frock of petals, wired
Bright blue, with silver wrappings round the stalks.
Sometimes I loved her: but I liked the smooth faces

Like the other mothers had, and told her so.
She laughed: she was never frightened: she took knocks
Square on the mouth, and wouldn't hit you back:
I never saw my mother dressed in black
But grief came . . . and she never let it go.

III

How do I know? What a fool question! Ask
How, sick of us, she wanted back herself
Too late: or ask in what mean arid way
Was snapped her pride. I only know, one day
Her eyes weren't tired, but weak; she still kept on
A while yet, till our frocks were out of school:
Poor old machine! I think it pricked a fool
Heart-deep, a million times; the clear white cloth,
That too; it tried to gather, as she told,
The running pleats; but something crumpled both . . .
Then swift sly hands smacked up from every task . . .
She was a cracked jug clinging to its shelf;
A fear, staring down at half-crossed Rubicon.

IV

But letting go . . . hands, eyes, teeth, body, all ways
A woman has of feeling proudly made . . .
Might still have left a dipping road; blue haze
(Kingfisher, sometimes), quilting soft afternoon;
But there were we, sprawled out: she was afraid,
Seeing us spring like mushrooms, big so soon;
Toadstools, perhaps she thought; her linen praise
God knows she earned; but hid it in her press,
Fearing to soil it with some bitterness
Against these young, who roared by different ways,
Drank new wine, breathed a different-seeming air;
Once she had liked her hands, but now no more
Her pride kept up its make in waist or hair:
Honour meant most. She listened by the door
For who'd betray it; but too spent to care.

Geoff Cochrane

Seven Hectic Takes

She's scornful; she's cross.
Or you hear in her laughter
the menace of sex.

You're rehearsing worship.
You're preparing a place in yourself.

You court her—none too bravely.
Give chocolates, a card.
You catch her wearing a sloppy pullover.

She's kind, capricious, lazy.
You're very aware of her bust;
you're all of a sudden aware
of her very breasty breasts.

'Visit. Ring. Do something.
Spare me your frivolous silence,' you write.
She unbuckles (you imagine) some Adonis.
Her fingers fastidiously weigh
cleft mauve tulip, balls.

And now, ah ha,
the fat brick wall of *nothing*,
of no further events—
beyond what *doesn't* happen
or happens only for *you*,
in *your* imagination.

Envoy

The sun comes up. The buses move.
A strange estrangement fills the weeks and months.
Do birds explain or bees apologise?
You remember her devoutly.

'There is chaos on the roads'

There is chaos on the roads.

It is winter in Khandallah;
It is winter in Kilbirnie.

Rain leaps in a spray
From streetlamp to streetlamp;
Wind gusts with a hoot through wires.

She doesn't want me, no,
But what do I do with her ghost,
That yellow hint of herself
She has failed to take with her?

There are wormholes in time.

There is darkness over an ocean.

Kevin Ireland

A Popular Romance

will you have me?
groaned the frog
my squashy love
is all agog

do you care?
complained the crab
a true heart serves
this horny scab

the prince exclaimed
if you agree
your love could change
the beast in me

they're all the same
the princess said
it's like a bestiary
in my bed

Peter Bland

The Bitch Madonna

In Tiepolo's
Woman Taken in Adultery
    Christ kneels
before this magnificent tart
    and looks
at Peter—who as usual
    wants to punch
some hypocrite on the nose.

    That look's a warning.
She's hot stuff. Don't blow it!
    With her around
someone has to throw stones.
    She laughs
at all this libido showing
    and stands
tit-proud. One bare shoulder

    daring anyone
to bruise *that* body. This mob
    —you can bet your bricks—
once offered other gifts. She

knows these well-heeled yobbos
intimately. Christ kneels . . .
          She probably thinks he's queer.
She prefers the fisherman

          he's holding back
with one mild-mannered glance.
          Her look is harder . . .
begging no one's pardon. After all
          it was always her job to bring
these bully-boys to the boil.
          she enjoys
watching the middle-classes rage

          as they try to disown
their dirty washing. Christ kneels—
          a mirror to the mob's deceit.
They stare back . . . eyes
          like broken bottles.
Tiepolo ejaculates on to his brush . . .
          body-colour
for his bitch madonna.

Marilyn Duckworth

Trap

Now that myself is trapped within your image
It matters little if you go or stay,
You only take what you already have,
What you already have you take away.

It is not you I love, it is that part
Of me which is submitted to your snare,
I nurse it as the rat his coming death,
Holding his breath and waiting to despair.

You lacked the cruelty, you lacked the skill
To lance my tenderness with borrowed knife,
But blundered on it with a casual hand
And trapped the larger pulses of my life.

And while myself is trapped within your image,
I notice you are changing separately,
That each grimace becomes a little altered,
Till you are gone who could have set me free.

Leprechaun Gold

Ten minutes' silence—mine—in a rented room,
While silk with sweat you choke like a stranded fish.
Suppose one day I am indiscreet enough
To break the prescribed silence, will you hear
Something as inescapable as death
Sliding its quicksilver into your ear?
No—for that ear is tuned only to words,
To 'love' and 'fond', to 'always' and to 'never'.
Words cannot break this silence circling close
Although your mouth surge to me like a river.

I picture you now in glittering leprechaun green,
Poised to snatch away the promised gold,
Grinning and spying out of puckered eyes
As from some gorse bush where you've chanced to hide
For half a lifespan.
I was warned of course, by you, of your mythical nature,
The invisibility cloak, the leprechaun wiles—
But lips and arms are easier to believe
Than sentences, and so I have breathed for miles
Running to your rainbow.

How shall I tell?
Your simple and most rare touchingness,
Which springs like a squirrel into my body's palm.
Your light bones plaited about me are as warm
As sunshine—are as soothing close as water,
Your mouth bleeds gold for fools to follow after.
And yet one day, you say, you will damage me
While I lie helpless, shaken with love as with laughter.

Norman Elder

Love-in-Idleness

Life is a habit, love's a habit, we
Lusting and lingering so fervently
Fondle from habit, and our clinging kiss
By frequent repetition, reaches this.

At my routine of loving do not curse,
Just thank your lucky stars it is no worse.

These formal incantations weave a mesh
To hold the foul beast from his meal of flesh.
He, too, is but a habit, something worn,
Of that high act from which a child is born.

Ruth Dallas

Song

Her true love has a second wife,
    Fair as she was fair,
Her love whom last she saw in grief,
    Who mourned for half a year,
Her gentle love who vowed her life
    Was sun to his and air.

In crystal that she would allow
    None but herself to choose,
Wine to pledge another vow
    Is raised to different eyes;
The cloth she hemmed is faded now,
    And none knows where she lies.

On Reading Love Poems

Gentle reader, do not
Spit, I pray, the pip
Of love's deep fruit,
The indigestible
Eyes that were her pearls,
Or let your ear be lulled
With all a triumphant tale.

Observe
Between the lines of Jack
In your own street
Not every Darby has his Joan.
At times recall
The basement room
Where Jill lives on.

Elizabeth Nannestad

The Witch Speaks Gently

Night of my imagining—

Where fish are running in the sea
and soft-bodied stars move
in all heaven's inhospitable grace
and winds feed on beaten grass
as wildfire in the hills
before the hills go down. Oh, my Dear
take me dancing.

I love to dance
as cold queens
long to die
laughing,
I like to dance
and this
is life
in life to me.

You, my silent and lonely hero of the hour,
you are my flower. My snapdragon.

He hardly replies. I
will not ask again.

Night of wild and easing sorrow. Night of reason.
Where now does your disappointment lie?

Somewhere in the night
a lover with dead white skin
lies breathing, thinking
I do not want to breathe again.

Your hips' hollow where you lie
is warm, and holds the smell
of salt and vinegar
like your skin, like mine.

You don't open those eyes.
Why not? You might as well.
There is no end to the number of times
the little death will come again.

Elizabeth Nannestad

Here We Go Again

I loved you as I love the light of morning
and leave you as I leave my stockings on the floor.

Everything is in some part yours, our things fill my room
and I am considerate. (Never before.)

What will there be here, when you're gone?

A bare page to write on.

A.R.P. Fairburn

The Woman to Her Lover

Had he battered me, called me whore,
had he thrust me out of door,
the end might have been different.
His kindness was deadly.
You ask me why, when the torrent came,
it was I who drowned and not he.
You do not understand.
You think emperors and great usurers are powerful.
Think of the power of the leprous beggar
who throws himself on the road and will not move.

I was defeated by pity,
the wooden horse that captures the iron city.

Anne French

Kitchens

Saturday morning on the kind of day
you don't recognise till afterwards
in my sister's kitchen, Pam wants
to know how I'm feeling. Like
an amputee in a minefield
too scared to move in any direction
I tell her, feeling the truth of it well
up in me as I say it, appalled, the telling
and the bloody stumps.

Do you miss him? Him
or the habits, like phantom
limb pain.

These questions, this unexpected
kindness. I didn't know what hit
me—just a false step I took
loving and believing regardless
of the evidence: the barbed wire
entanglements, the limping survivors
asking after each other in kitchens.

James K. Baxter

from *Pig Island Letters*

2

From an old house shaded with macrocarpas
Rises my malady.
Love is not valued much in Pig Island
Though we admire its walking parody,

That brisk gaunt woman in the kitchen
Feeding the coal range, sullen
To all strangers, lest one should be
Her antique horn-red Satan.

Her man, much baffled, grousing in the pub,
Discusses sales
Of yearling lambs, the timber in a tree
Thrown down by autumn gales,

Her daughter, reading in her room
A catalogue of dresses,
Can drive a tractor, goes to Training College,
Will vote on the side of the Bosses,

Her son is moodier, has seen
An angel with a sword
Standing above the clump of old man manuka
Just waiting for the word

To overturn the cities and the rivers
And split the house like a rotten totara log.
Quite unconcerned he sets his traps for possums
And whistles to his dog.

The man who talks to the masters of Pig Island
About the love they dread
Plaits ropes of sand, yet I was born among them
And will lie some day with their dead.

Vincent O'Sullivan

July, July

There's a dreary morning coming up,
the sky's as dull as a shoe.
It'll be a day that won't touch
even the last gasp of blue.

The best words won't work—
love and the rest, love
and the glint it's meant to give,
love's as slack as an old glove.

The harbour lies there meek
in a window looking south,
the south and its imagined fangs
in that imagined mouth.

'That'll be the day' as we like
to say, but it won't be today,
'There's a dreary week of it coming up,'
is what we say, and say.

Yet a day when you don't expect it,
sheer glitter ringing about
as if all the cutlery drawers of Kelburn
had been tipped out,

a day when the knives don't nick,
when the dry horizons scale.
There's a shine and flicker to the wind,
southern rancours fail

to cut the ice we expect,
the mountains ride their horses
with their withers of snow,
and the wind, the stroked manes of the horses.

C.K. Stead

After the Wedding

1

After the wedding comparing notes with
Cousin Elspeth and Cousin Caroline
about our childhood bareback riding
on the Kaiwaka farm—

        How, fallen with your
10-year legs, did you get back up
even supposing he stood for you?

Cousin E remembered vaulting from the back
of her pet pig.
        I used the ruts worn deep
by the cream sledge—stood him in the hollow
and leapt from its edge.

        Elspeth
and her sister, blond babies
under the trees I climbed—

        wooden verandah
hot dry garden sheltered by macrocarpa
dogs panting in shade
        my face black
from the summer burn-off.

2

In sleep I still trace those tracks
below gum trees
        skirting the swamp
through bush to that pool of pools
where the small brown fish suspend themselves
in shafts of light.
        My feet sink
midstream in heaped silt
clouding the flow.

        Water had cut its way
through black rock greened with moss
down to that glassy stillness overhung
with trees.

In the rock cleft
a deep hole water-worn and cold and dark—

I caught the eel that lived there
        its sinuous spirit.

3

In recollection summer is forever
renewing itself even in the thickest
leafmould shade.
           It draws a life
from heat in the ploughed field
where I gathered fossil gum
               or in the hayfield
or in sunlight above the flame
above the dam.

        Cousin Elspeth, Cousin Caroline
cantered bareback
                  fell
(years after me) from the same horse.

4

Weddings are full of God and the word of God
and the word God. I wonder what they mean.
To be one with your body, your body one with the world—
more than a marriage, it's a consummation
bracken and oil-flame like red cellophane
flapping on the hill-slope.
                Eden
won't ask you back, you must make your way
in dreams, by moonlight, or by the broad light of day.

5

There was another stream, a creek
on the far side of the road
where the old house had been.
        It ran through reeds
silent.

The moons repeat themselves
the moreporks retort
the eel and its sibilants
are fluent

      an old chimney stands.

6

It's not what the landscape says
but the way it's said which is a
richness of saying, even of the thing
said—

      that finely articulated slope
a few words at the water
the breathy manuka and the precise
pernickity ti tree

    a long last sentence of cloud
struck out by the dark.

After the wedding
I lie in darkness
I see something that might be myself
        step out for a moment.

It makes the moon
look at itself in water
       it makes the stars
gaze.
     It hears a nightbird and something
        that rustles
in reeds.

It sees itself called
       to light up a silent
vast
    beautiful
        indifferent

waste—

mirror to the mystery
mirrored.

7

Break it
    (the mirror)

the Supreme Intelligence
is always silent
       and death will come
in the guise of just this stillness
or another

      but that was always the case.

8

'Marriages are made in Heaven'
                              —not so.

We marry to be nearer the earth
cousins of the fur and stalk
                          talking together

that brown water reflecting
those green hills.

Bill Manhire

Jalopy: The End of Love

Do you drive an old car?
Or a jalopy?
Now where could that word come from?

Somewhere in the world
someone you know
must be driving a jalopy.

As for you, one day you are out
on a country road
miles from the sort of place

that might be miles from anywhere
and your car breaks down.
Well, it's an old car.

And somewhere in the world
someone you used to love
has that ancient photograph of you

sitting behind the wheel
high on the Coromandel.
It's a jalopy.

Just at the moment though
it doesn't want to start.
Whatever it is, it's finished.

Robert Sullivan

from *Tai Tokerau Poems*

6 *This Much is True*

Watching a cockatoo in its cage reminds me of my position,
I must go back to the Bay of Islands, get out of the city.

I've lived here all my life—loved, almost died, been sent away
and returned for more. But I don't know how I'll survive this.

Tonight the sweet devil's got my soul. It drives me crazy.
You're a real rhythm kid, such a fine young cannibal, on the floor

of Candyo's rubbing the rose—which has a thorn like your woman's
scorn. Our hearts lie close together yet our bodies don't.

We do what we should, wishing what we shouldn't. So I sit outside
your door, whistling at a bloody cockatoo, wondering when you'll

let me off the hook. I've really had it, this isn't love!
What have I done to deserve it, Kim? leaving me in the eye
                    of the needle, a thread without a stitch.

A.R.D. Fairburn

Night Song

Though Time's black mountain overhangs
the night where she's engrossed in sleep
its shadow cannot bruise my love,
so calm she lies, she dreams so deep.

She is not hurt by what shall be,
death stands enchanted in her eyes;
remote and lovely, a floating flower
on the lily pool of sleep she lies.

Dream deep, my love, as in the time
when your sweet spirit was unborn,
but rise up when the east is purple
and dress your hair for Judgment morn.

Lauris Edmond

from *Wellington Letter*

II

You are the smiling photo beside
the telephone, the laughter stilled
on a tape casually recorded. There are
other exact presences; it's true death's
winter passes, we meet in a new spring
and I walk your green aisles of silence
in a remembered confiding. In four years
I have given up straining, have learned

to stand still, unprotesting as forlorn
couples do when the train's gone, taking
a child to the dangerous city. Through
breaking clouds I see there was a true
madness in you—'I'll eat a lily' only
you could say, and laugh, and do it
despite expostulations; poisonous?
You didn't care, taking yourself too
lightly even then. Four years. It's
hardly time, yet this is the work
grief gives, to set about composing
the lifetime that we thought we knew,
without falsity or fear to try to make
it whole. One remains accountable.

Death's an explosion in the mine
of love; this letter tells of
reconstruction, failed attempts,
of gifts, of visitations from those
who come like neighbours bringing
soup and clothes to families made
homeless by disaster; so love
returns, limps in, is recognised.

VIII

'Let's discover pub talk' the young poet
pronounced, 'not to set ourselves apart . . .'
Well, it was all there, the carpet thick
with beer, the juke box hollering, a little

joker no one knew coming and going with
the mild and muddied bonhomie of booze—
a good fellow without doubt but I think,
poet, he doesn't want to be romanticised.

Yet I admit we proved some point about
the place, four of us attending to those
two—good men, respectful, never close
till now—while they told tales of work
and friends, theories, mistakes and
passionate misconceptions; a touch solemn
(that was the beer), certainly excessive;
it was a subtle, risky sharing, abandoned
yet more watchful than it looked. Listening
I thought of old and common voices; was it
thus, perhaps, the dialogue that asked
around for truth (the elusive comrade)
while laurel sticks were doodling in
the hot Athenian dust?

                                Then they embraced,
laughing crazily, and you could see that
every one of us was drunk with love.

XVIII

Dear and gentle ghost, I have come
to an end; and did not find, as
perhaps I hoped, that you would speak
again if we could find the words.
Rather I know that though love's sick
body is restored by love there is none
great enough to cross the seas that roar
between our separate mountain tops.
We embark; there is no arriving.

You have your choice, I mine; and soon
we shall both be one with the constant
earth, the tides that put out to
the hurting uncertain future; strange
gods will brood above our sleep of
clay, their voices echo through us
where we lie, change, dissolve,
take on new lives. We are the cells
of time; snow will fall upon us
with its crisping touch, wind blow

our dust, water wash us in the pebbled
body of the sea, and the stars
take always their dark road.

Our words will be lost but our love
will enter the life of the land
like the dust a sunset lights up
with its recurring fire. Now the sky
broadens, sun touches the water.
I tell you it will be a fine day.

Vincent O'Sullivan

Elegy: Again

You are on a railway platform
in the driest country we had ever seen.
We stand in the heat by a row of shagged
pot plants and I think how green

was always the colour as you came to mind,
a green coat once by a corner in Florence
when you didn't see me, leaning towards a match.
You are ten yards away and ah, the distance,

even then; or our lying side by side,
your hair that I joked was like a fire
stalking a step behind you, a smokey
brilliance even now, when words like 'desire'

are husks, shells, dead tongues,
as once we reached them down from the living
tree, the green sky, and our hands
brushing like something scorched, loving

without the palaver of having to say.
And the utter ashes of it now, the same
as if I'd read about someone else, un-
moved. And you, caged in freedoms beyond flame.

K.O. Arvidson

from *The Four Last Songs of Richard Strauss at Takahe Creek above the Kaipara*

2 *September*

(Hesse)

I am assembled here, at ease
in foreboding. I have measured the shadow
dying, and the brilliant wind
is alive with new things, lambs and petals and light,
asserting permanence. And yet,
this little thrush, that madly
flew through the scents of newness, now
grows cold within my hand. Strange noon,
to smite so casually, to freeze so small a thing
and drop it on warm grass!
I watched this little bird. It sped like a thistle
recklessly, bucketing on the air,
and very loud: implying, I think,
mortality, because I watched it all the way
from the long soft grass through that abandonment
to the tree so landmark-large, to the last and sudden
blindness, staggering ecstasy, light
singing
    death.

      I am assembled here, at ease
in foreboding. And my desire?
My love should bury this with love.

My love would not. My love would
toss it in the air.

3 *Im Abendrot*

(von Eichendorff)

The far Brynderwyns heave across the harbour,
rising above the second tide, mountains
in mangrove moving, weaving
the last complexities of the sun. These
are a tangle of reflections. Over them,

the next peninsula shines yellow,
pastoral century of slow change,
and the roofs of pioneers, like beacons, prophesy
the imminence of fishermen, their lights
alive and casting, quick
to be out before the strong tide sucks and runs.

    I sing of our long voyaging,
    and you who led me, at my side;
    I sing the saddest of all things;
    I sing the unaccomplished bride.

The hills will cease to float soon, and the mangroves
ripple themselves away.
The wandering flames of grass will calm, and the cattle
boom night's gullies up and down. My lights
will anchor a headland. Boats will take bearings,
seeking the channel; and then,
the Kaipara will move out.
A shag clap-claps in shallows.
I point the way to an open sea,
though all my doors are closed,
and I within.

    Go slowly, sun. A gentle death
    of day is in the birds that wheel
    in clouds to their accustomed rest,
    and in the racing of the keel

    before the racing of the tide,
    and in the crowding of dark trees.
    I sing the unaccomplished bride.
    I sing my death in all of these.

Sources

The editor and publisher would like to thank copyright holders for permission to reproduce copyright material. Every effort has been made to trace the original source of all material contained in this book. Where the attempt has been unsuccessful the editor and publisher would be pleased to hear from the author or publisher concerned to rectify any omission.

Fleur Adcock, 'Afterwards' and 'Happy Ending', *High Tide in the Garden*, OUP, London, 1971; 'An Illustration to Dante', 'Tokens', and 'Folie à Deux', *The Scenic Route*, OUP, London, 1974; 'Ancestor to Devotee', *Looking Back*, OUP, London, 1997; 'Double-Take', *The Incident Book*, OUP, Oxford, 1986; 'The Lover', *The Eye of the Hurricane*, A.H. & A.W. Reed, Wellington, Auckland, 1964. **John Allison**, 'In/Fidelities', *Dividing the Light*, Hazard Press, Christchurch, 1997. **Mohammad Amir**, 'Love', *Kapiti Poems 7*, Rawhiti Press, Pukera Bay, in association with Whitireia Publishing, Porirua, and Daphne Brasell Associates Press, Wellington, 1994. **K.O. Arvidson**, 'By the Clear Fountain', 'Riding the Pendulum', and 'September' and 'Im Abendrot' from 'The Four Last Songs of Richard Strauss at Takahe Creek above the Kaipara', *Riding the Pendulum: Poems 1961–69*, OUP, Wellington, 1973. **John Barr**, 'Meet Me When the Moon is Up' and 'The Bachelor's Resolve', *Poems and Songs*, John Greig & Son, Edinburgh, 1860. **B.E. Baughan**, from 'The Paddock': extract from 'Song of the White Clover', *Shingle-Short and Other Verses*, Whitcombe & Tombs, Christchurch, 1908. **James K. Baxter**, from 'Pig Island Letters' (2), 'At the Fox Glacier Hotel', 'Mill Girl', 'On the Death of Her Body', 'My Love Late Walking', and 'He Waiata Mo Te Kare', *Collected Poems* (ed. John Weir), OUP, Wellington, 1980; 'Let Time be Still', *The Rock Woman: Selected Poems*, OUP, Oxford, 1969. **J.C. Beaglehole**, 'You were Standing', *Rata: New Zealand Annual*, Wellington, 1932. **James Bertram**, 'To Charles Brasch at Sixty', *Occasional Verses*, Wai-te-Ata Press, Wellington, 1971. **Ursula Bethell**, from 'Six Memorials': 'October 1935', *Collected Poems* (ed. Vincent O'Sullivan), VUP, 1985 (new edn 1997). **Tony Beyer**, 'Losing You', *Brute Music*, Hard Echo Press, Auckland, 1984; 'The Ornamentalists', *The Singing Ground: Poems*, Caxton Press, Christchurch, 1986. **Peter Bland**, 'Bear Dance', *Selected Poems*, John McIndoe, Dunedin, 1987; 'Settling Down', *The Man with the Carpet-Bag*, Caxton Press, Christchurch, 1972; 'The Bitch Madonna', *Stone Tents*, London Magazine Editions, London, 1981. **Jenny Bornholdt**, 'The Boyfriends', 'The Loved One', 'In Love', and 'Wedding Song', *Miss New Zealand: Selected Poems*, VUP, 1997; 'Lake Rotoiti', *How We Met*, VUP, 1995. **Charles Brasch**, 'In Your Presence', *Collected Poems* (ed. Alan Roddick), OUP, Auckland, 1984; 'To C.H. Roberts', *Disputed Ground: Poems 1939–45*, Caxton Press, Christchurch, 1948. **Betty Bremner**, 'Versions', *The Scarlet Runners*, Rawhide Press,

Pukerua Bay, 1991. **Erick Brenstrum**, 'First Love', *Thalassa: The Words of the Dream. Poems 1971–81*, Breath Press, Wellington, 1981; 'Wave-runner', previously unpublished. **Bub Bridger**, 'Confession' and 'Love Poem', *Up There on the Hill*, Mallinson Rendel, Wellington, 1989. **James Brown**, 'A New Position' and 'Map Reference', *Go Round Power Please*, VUP, 1995. **Rachel Bush**, 'You Wouldn't Read About It', *The Hungry Woman*, VUP, 1997. **Kate Camp**, 'Dear Sir' and 'In Your Absence', *Unfamiliar Legends of the Stars*, VUP, 1998. **Alistair Te Ariki Campbell**, 'August' and 'Lament', *Wild Honey*, OUP, London, 1964; 'Love Song for Meg' and 'Why Don't You Talk to Me?', *Kapiti: Selected Poems 1947–71*, Pegasus Press, Christchurch, 1972; 'To My Grandson Oliver Maireriki Aged One Day', *Stone Rain: The Polynesian Strain*, Hazard Press, Christchurch, 1992; 'Bon Voyage', *Pocket Collected Poems*, Hazard Press, Christchurch, 1996. **Meg Campbell**, 'After Loving', 'The Way Back', and 'This Morning at Dawn', *The Way Back*, Te Kotare Press, Pukerua Bay, 1981; 'Sea Creatures', *A Durable Fire*, Te Kotare Press, Pukerua Bay, 1982; from 'A Diary 79', *Orpheus and Other Poems*, Te Kotare Press, Pukerua Bay, 1990. **Gordon Challis**, 'Poem for Magda', *Building*, Caxton Press, Christchurch, 1963. **Geoff Cochrane**, 'Seven Hectic Takes' and 'There is chaos on the roads', *Into India*, VUP, 1999. **Allen Curnow**, 'A Woman in Mind', *Collected Poems 1933–73*, A.H. & A.W. Reed, Wellington, 1974 (first appeared in *Enemies: Poems 1934–36*, Caxton Press, Christchurch, 1937). **Ruth Dallas**, 'A Girl's Song', 'Song', 'On Reading Love Poems', and 'Tinker, Tailor', *Country Road and Other Poems, 1947–52*, Caxton Press, Christchurch, 1953. **Basil Dowling**, 'The Best of All', *Canterbury and Other Poems*, Caxton Press, Christchurch, 1949. **Charles Doyle**, 'My Love Lies Down Tonight', *Distances*, Paul's Book Arcade, Auckland, 1963. **Marilyn Duckworth**, 'Trap' and 'Leprechaun Gold', *Other Lovers' Children*, Pegasus Press, Christchurch, 1975. **Eileen Duggan**, 'The Boastful Lover', 'The Bushfeller' (the latter originally from *Poems 1937–39*), and 'The Tides Run Up the Wairau', *Selected Poems* (ed. Peter Whiteford), VUP, 1994. **Peggy Dunstan**, 'Even in Sleep', *A Particular Deep*, Pegasus Press, Christchurch, 1974; 'Looking Back', *Patterns on Glass*, Pegasus Press, Christchurch, 1968. **Lauris Edmond**, 'A Reckoning', 'Demande de Midi', 'Doubletake', 'Epithalamion', 'Late Starling', 'Learning to Ride', 'The Names', 'Those Roses', and from 'Wellington Letter': III, VIII, XVIII, *Selected Poems 1975–94*, Bridget Williams Books, Wellington, 1994; 'Spring Afternoon, Dunedin', *A Matter of Timing*, AUP, 1996. **Murray Edmond**, 'Go to Woe', *From the Word Go*, AUP, 1992. **Norman Elder**, 'Love-in-a-Mist' and 'Love-in-Idleness', *Verse*, self-published [Hart Print, Hastings, NZ], 1965. **Wilhelmina Sherriff Elliott**, 'Nga Huia', *From Zealandia: A Book of Verse*, John M. Watkins, London, 1925. **A.R.D. Fairburn**, 'Night Song' and 'Winter Night', *Selected Poems* (ed. Mac Jackson), VUP, 1995; 'Poem', 'A Farewell', and 'The Woman to Her Lover', *Collected Poems* (ed. Denis Glover), Pegasus Press, Christchurch, 1966. **Fiona Farrell**, 'Jigsaw' and 'Love Songs: Seven Wishes, Full Spring', *Cutting Out*, AUP, 1987. **Anne French**, 'Boys' Night Out', 'Kitchens', and 'Parallel Universes', *Boys' Night Out*, AUP, 1998;

'Collisions', *All Cretans are Liars*, AUP, 1987; from 'Two Love Poems': I and 'New Zealanders at Home', *Seven Days on Mykonos*, AUP, 1993; 'Three Love Poems', *Cabin Fever*, AUP, 1990. **Kathleen Gallagher**, 'I Love You Annie', *Tara*, Nag's Head Press, Christchurch, 1987. **Ruth Gilbert**, 'Even in the Dark' and 'Green Hammock, White Magnolia Tree', *Collected Poems*, Black Robin, Wellington, 1984; 'Rachel', *Lazarus and Other Poems*, A.H. & A.W. Reed, Wellington, 1949. **Denis Glover**, 'Afterthought', *Enter Without Knocking: Selected Poems*, Pegasus Press, Christchurch, 1971; 'In Needless Doubt', 'The Two Flowers', and 'Brightness', *Denis Glover: Selected Poems* (ed. Bill Manhire), VUP, 1995; 'I'm an Odd Fish', *Dancing to My Tune*, Catspaw Press, Wellington, 1974. **Kathleen Grattan**, 'A Sudden Radiance', *The Music of What Happens*, Writers & Artists Press, Auckland, 1987. **Russell Haley**, 'Tannery Hill' and 'The Dogs/The Face', *On the Fault Line*, Hawk Press, Paraparaumu, 1977. **Bernadette Hall**, 'Amica', *An Anthology of New Zealand Poetry in English* (ed. J. Bornholdt, G. O'Brien, and M. Williams), OUP, Auckland, 1997; 'Duck' and 'Lovesong', *Still Talking*, VUP, 1997. **Michael Harlow**, from 'Poem Then, for Love' and 'Only on the White', *Vlaminck's Tie*, AUP/OUP, Auckland, 1985. **William Hart-Smith**, 'Smoke Signal' and 'Postage Stamp', *Selected Poems 1936–84* (ed. Brian Dibble), Angus & Robertson, Sydney, 1985. **Dinah Hawken**, 'A Friend', *Small Stories of Devotion*, VUP, 1991; (Meeting on the Tideline) from 'Water, Women & Birds Gather', *Water, Leaves, Stones*, VUP, 1995. **Robin Healey**, 'Night Kitchen' and 'Pullover', *Night Kitchen*, Mallinson Rendel, Wellington, 1985. **J.R. Hervey**, 'Even So Came Love', *Selected Poems*, Caxton Press, Christchurch, 1940; 'She was My Love Who Could Deliver', *She was My Spring*, Caxton Press, Christchurch, 1954. **David Howard**, from 'The Last Word', 3, *Head First*, Hard Echo Press, Auckland, 1985. **Sam Hunt**, 'A Long Time' and 'August Steam', *Collected Poems 1963–80*, Penguin Books, Auckland, 1980; 'Bottle to Battle to Death', *Selected Poems*, Penguin Books, Auckland, 1987; 'Cuckold Song' and 'Those Eyes; Such Mist', *Drunkard's Garden*, Hampson Hunt, Wellington, 1977; 'Stabat Mater', *South into Winter: Poems and Roadsongs*, Alister Taylor, Wellington, 1973. **Jan Hutchison**, 'A Lesson on the Beach', 'Laura Sings to Her Corn-Cob Doll', and 'My Mother and Father', *The Long Sleep is Over*, Steele Roberts, Aotearoa, NZ, 1999. **Robin Hyde**, 'Escape'; from 'The People': II, III and IV; and from 'Houses by the Sea': 'The Beaches' vi, *Selected Poems* (ed. Lydia Wevers), OUP, Auckland, 1984; 'Silence', *The Desolate Star and Other Poems*, Whitcombe & Tombs Ltd, Christchurch, 1929; from 'Journey from New Zealand'. **Kevin Ireland**, 'A Popular Romance', *Educating the Body*, Caxton Press, Christchurch, 1967; 'A Way of Sorrow' and 'Establishing the Facts', *Orchids, Hummingbirds and Other Poems*, AUP/OUP, 1974; 'The Professor of Love', *Practice Night in the Drill Hall*, OUP, Wellington, 1984. **Michael Jackson**, 'A Marriage', 'Fille de Joie: Congo', and 'Parentage', *Latitudes of Exile*, John McIndoe, Dunedin, 1976; from 'Fragments', i, and 'Seven Mysteries', *Going On*, John McIndoe, Dunedin, 1985. **Helen Jacobs**, 'The Ice of Kindness', *Pools over Stone*, Sudden Valley Press, Christchurch, 1995.

Adrienne Jansen, 'A Poem of Farewell' and 'Connections', previously unpublished. **Andrew Johnson**, 'In White', *The Sounds*, VUP, 1996. **Louis Johnson**, 'Dirge', *The Sun Among the Ruins*, Pegasus Press, Christchurch, 1951; 'Remainders' and 'Nisi', *Winter Apples*, Mallinson Rendel, Wellington, 1984; 'Statistics', *Last Poems* (ed. P. Bland and T. Sturm), Antipodes Press, Wellington, 1990; 'Summer Sunday', *Fires and Patterns*, Jacaranda Press, Brisbane, 1975. **M.K. Joseph**, 'Cinderella', 'For My Children', 'Girl, Boy, Flower, Bicycle', 'The Girl Who Stayed at Home', and 'Romeo and Juliet (Duet)', *Inscription on a Paper Dart: Selected Poems 1945–72*, AUP/OUP, 1974. **Jan Kemp**, poem ('A puriri moth's wing') and poem ('It was your face'), *Against the Softness of Women*, Caveman Press, Dunedin, 1976. **Fiona Kidman**, 'Earth- quake Weather' (from *On the Tightrope*), 'Pact for Mother & Teenager', and 'Wakeful Nights' 3, 4, 5, 6, *Wakeful Nights: Poems Selected and New*, Vintage, Auckland, 1991; 'The Blue Dress', *Going to the Chathams: Poems 1977–84*, Heinemann Publishers, Auckland, 1985. **Koenraad Kuiper**, from 'Addresses': II 'To His Mistress', *Mikrokosmos*, One Eyed Press, Otaki, 1990. **Leonard Lambert**, 'Cold Eyes', 'My Early Love', and 'The Lovers at Sixty', *A Washday Romance Poems: 1969–79*, John McIndoe, Dunedin, 1980. **Hugh Lauder**, 'Silence' and 'The Descent', *Over the White Wall*, Caxton Press, Christchurch, 1985. **Michele Leggott**, 'Dear Heart', *Swimmers, Dancers*, AUP, 1991; 'Keep- ing Warm', *DIA*, AUP, 1994. **Iain Lonie**, 'A Postcard of Cornwall', *Courting Death*, Wai-te-ata Press, Wellington, 1984; 'Mirror Language', *Winter Walk at Morning*, VUP, 1991. **Bill Manhire**, 'Children', 'Love Poem', Poem ('When we touch'), 'The Proof', 'The Elaboration', 'The Kiss', 'City Life', *Sheet Music: Poems 1967–82*, VUP, 1996; 'Jalopy: The End of Love', *Milky Way Bar*, VUP, 1991; 'My Sunshine', *My Sunshine*, VUP, 1996. **Katherine Mansfield**, 'He Wrote' and 'The Meeting', *Poems of Katherine Mansfield* (ed. Vincent O'Sullivan), OUP, London, 1988. **R.A.K. Mason**, 'Thigh to Thigh', 'Our Love was a Grim Citadel', 'Lugete o Veneres', and 'Footnote to John ii 4', *Collected Poems, 1905–71*, Pegasus Press, Christchurch, 1975; 'Flow at Full Moon', *This Dark will Lighten: Selected Poems 1923–41*, Caxton Press, Christchurch, 1941. **Rachel McAlpine**, 'Before the Fall', 'How to Live Without Love', and 'Zig-Zag up a Thistle', *Recording Angel*, Mallinson Rendel, Wellington, 1983. **Gary McCormick**, 'Time', *Lost at Sea*, Hodder Moa Beckett, Auckland, 1995. **Donald McDonald**, 'Time', *Sidi Reszegh and Other Verses*, Progressive Publishing Society, Wellington, 1944. **Cilla McQueen**, 'A Lightning Tree', 'Wild Sweets', 'Wham Bananaskin Catapult', and 'Crikey', *Wild Sweets*, John McIndoe, Dunedin, 1986. **Harvey McQueen**, 'To Anne' and 'At Ease', *Oasis Motel and Other Poems*, Black Robin Press, Wellington, 1986. **Heather McPherson**, 'A Money-Bean Tree' and 'Be Quiet', *The Third Myth*, Tauranga Moana Press, Tauranga, 1986. **Don McRae**, 'My Love', *The Coal is Red: Poems about Mining People and Others*, self-published, Auckland, 1981. **Michael Mor- rissey**, 'Movie Madonnas', *She's Not the Child of Sylvia Plath*, Sword Press, Christchurch, 1981. **Martha Morseth**, 'Broken Porcelain', *Catching the Rainbow*, New Zealand Poetry, Wellington, 1996. **Elizabeth Nannestad**, 'La

Strada', 'On Love', 'The Kiss', and 'Against Housework', *If He's a Good Dog He'll Swim*, AUP, 1996; 'The Witch Speaks Gently', 'Here We Go Again', 'We Watched the Moon Rise', and 'You Must be Joking', *Jump*, AUP, 1986. **James Norcliffe**, 'Easy Thai Cooking' and 'In the Food Court', *A Kind of Kingdom*, VUP, 1998. **Gregory O'Brien**, 'Tall Woman Story II', *Winter I Was*, VUP, 1999. **W.H. Oliver**, 'A Performance of *Death and the Maiden*', *Fire without Phoenix*, Caxton Press, Christchurch, 1957; 'Peacocks' and 'The Swineherd', *Out of Season*, OUP, Wellington, 1980. **Bob Orr**, 'Signatures', *Poems for Moira*, Hawk Press, Eastbourne, NZ, 1979; 'Sugar Boat' and 'Love Poem', *Cargo*, Voice Press, Wellington, 1983. **Vincent O'Sullivan**, 'Elegy, of Sorts' and 'July, July', *Seeing You Asked*, VUP, 1998; 'Elegy: Again', previously unpublished. **Alistair Paterson**, from 'What Never Happened' 5, 'Jennie Roache Love All the Boys in the World', *Birds Flying*, Pegasus Press, Christchurch, 1973. **Patuwhakairi**, 'Lament for Ngaro' (trans. Margaret Orbell), *Poetry Yearbook*, vol. 5 (ed. F. McKay), John McIndoe, Dunedin, 1982. **Vivienne Plumb**, 'Before the Operation', 'I Love Those Photos', 'Journey to the Centre', and 'Women Often Dream of Flying', *Salamanca*, HeadworX, Wellington, 1998. **Roma Potiki**, 'Incognito', *Shaking the Tree*, Steele Roberts, Wellington, 1998. **Sarah Quigley**, 'Anglo-Indian Summer', *AUP New Poets I*, AUP, 1999. **Laura Ranger**, 'Mum', *Laura's Poems*, Godwit Press, Auckland, 1995. **Alan Riach**, 'A Poem about Four Feet', 'Necessity of Listening', and 'That Silence', *First and Last Songs*, AUP, 1995. **Harry Ricketts**, 'How Things Are' and 'Under the Radar', *Nothing to Declare*, HeadworX, Wellington, 1998. **Bill Sewell**, 'Aubade', *Making the Far Land Glow*, John McIndoe, Dunedin, 1986; 'Bread and Wine', previously unpublished. **Iain Sharp**, 'Owed to Joy', *Printout 12*, Auckland, 1997; 'The Plan', *Printout 8*, Auckland, 1994; 'The Constitution' and 'Watching the Motorway by Moonlight', *The Pierrot Variations*, Hard Echo Press, Auckland, 1985. **Keith Sinclair**, 'A Night Full of Nothing', 'Fathers and Sons Night', 'The Furies', 'Girl Loved by the Moon', and 'To Her for Christmas', *Moontalk: Poems New and Selected*, AUP, 1993; 'The Lovers', *Strangers or Beasts*, Caxton Press, Christchurch, 1954. **Elizabeth Smither**, 'A Cortège of Daughters', 'St Paul's Kind of Love', 'The Lions', 'Temptations of St Antony by His Housekeeper', *The Tudor Style: Poems New and Selected*, AUP, 1993; 'To Write of Love', *Here Come the Clouds*, Alister Taylor, Wellington, 1975. **Kendrick Smithyman**, 'Ambush', *Auto/Biographies*, AUP, 1992; 'Could You Once Regain', *An Anthology of New Zealand Verse* (ed. Robert Chapman and Jonathon Bennett), OUP, London and Wellington, 1956; 'Kingfisher Song' and 'This Blonde Girl', *Selected Poems* (ed. Peter Simpson), AUP, 1989; 'Still Life', *Dwarf with a Billiard Cue*, AUP/OUP, 1978. **Brent Southgate**, 'Windfalls' and 'The Disappearance', *Participants and Others*, Amphedesma Press, London, 1970; 'Tactics', *Poetry New Zealand*, vol. 3 (ed. Frank McKay), Pegasus Press, Christchurch, 1976. **Charles Spear**, 'Audrey', *Twopence Coloured*, Caxton Press, Christchurch, 1951. **Elizabeth Spencer**, 'Wife in Wartime', *Private Gardens: An Anthology of New Zealand Women Poets* (ed. Reimke Ensing), Caveman Press, Dunedin, 1977. **Mary Stanley**, 'Per Diem et per Noctem',

Starveling Year and Other Poems, AUP, 1994. **C.K. Stead**, from 'Quesada', 1, *Quesada: Poems 1972–74*, The Shed, Auckland, 1975; 'Tall Girl' (from 'Four Harmonics of Regret'), *Whether the Will is Free: Poems 1954–62*, Paul's Book Arcade, Auckland, 1964; from 'From the Clodian Songbook', 2, and from 'After the Wedding', *Between*, AUP, 1988. **J.C. Sturm**, 'Before Dawn, Before Dark' and 'Maori to Pakeha', *Dedications*, Steele Roberts & Associates, Wellington, 1997. **Robert Sullivan**, from 'Community Poems: 4 Hand that Stilled the Water' and from 'Tai Tokerau Poems': 6 'This Much is True', *Jazz Waiata*, AUP, 1990. **John Summers**, 'Bush Lawyer', *Prancing Before the Ark*, printed at Caxton Press, Pisces Print [sic], Christchurch, 1982. **George Sweet**, 'The Shopping List', previously unpublished. **Brian Turner**, 'Shining', *All that Blue Can Be*, John McIndoe, Dunedin, 1989; 'Taking It as It Comes', *Bones*, John McIndoe, Dunedin, 1985; 'Wife', *New Zealand Love Poems* (ed. John Bertram), John McIndoe, Dunedin, 1977. **Hone Tuwhare**, 'Love Pome', 'Annie', 'In October, Mary Quite Contemporary will be Seven Months Gone', 'Lovers', and 'Mad', *Mihi: Collected Poems*, Penguin Books, Auckland, 1987; 'You have to Come First Before You Can Go' and 'Humming', *Short Back and Sideways: Poems and Prose*, Godwit Press, Auckland, 1992; 'Yes' and 'When the Karaka Trees Whistled and Said to Us: Kia Kaha!', from *Shape-shifter*, Steele Roberts, Wellington, 1997. **Anton Vogt**, 'Marriage', *Poems for a War*, Progressive Publishing Society, Wellington 1943; 'For a Child's Drawing', *Nowhere Far from the Sea: An Anthology of New Zealand Verse*, Whitcombe & Tombs, Christchurch, 1971. **Ian Wedde**, 'The Arrangement' and 'Sonnet for Carlos', '2 for Rose', and 'It's Time' (the last three from 'Earthly: Sonnets for Carlos'), *Driving into the Storm: Selected Poems*, OUP, Auckland, 1987; 'Drought', *Spells for Coming Out*, AUP/OUP, 1977; 'Homecoming', *Made Over*, Stephen Chan, Auckland, 1974; 'Beautiful Gold Girl of the Sixties', *Georgicon*, VUP, 1984. **Albert Wendt**, 'My Mother Dances', *Shaman of Visions,* AUP/OUP, 1984. **Nick Williamson**, 'Making Love', previously unpublished. **Pat Wilson**, 'The Farewell', *The Bright Sea*, Pegasus Press, Christchurch, 1950.

AUP = Auckland University Press, Auckland; OUP = Oxford University Press; VUP = Victoria University Press, Wellington.

Index of First Lines

Index of Poets and Titles